The End of Medicine
and the
Last Doctor

*Dedicated to Scott and Thomas
and their generation*

The End of Medicine

and the

Last Doctor

Sidney Lowry

Emeritus Professor
Physicist and Physician

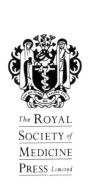

The ROYAL
SOCIETY of
MEDICINE
PRESS Limited

Published by the Royal Society of Medicine Press Ltd
1 Wimpole Street, London W1G 0AE, UK
Tel: +44 (0)20 7290 2921
Fax: +44 (0)20 7290 2929
E-mail: publishing@rsm.ac.uk
Website: www.rsmpress.co.uk

British Library Cataloguing in Publication Data
A catalogue record for this book is available from the British Library

---

ISBN 978-1-85315-967-1

Distribution in Europe and Rest of World:

Marston Book Services Ltd
PO Box 269
Abingdon
Oxon OX14 4YN, UK
Tel:+44 (0)1235 465 500
Fax: +44 (0)1235 465 555
Email: direct.order@marston.com

Distribution in the USA and Canada:
Royal Society of Medicine Press Ltd
c/o BookMasters, Inc
30 Amberwood Parkway
Ashland, Ohio 44805, USA
Tel: +1 800 247 6553 / +1 800 266 5564
Fax: +1 419 281 6883
Email: order@bookmasters.com

Typeset by Phoenix Photosetting, Chatham, Kent, UK
Printed and bound in India by Replika Press Pvt. Ltd.

Contents

Preface

I have borrowed the idea for the title of this book from Francis Fukuyama's *The End of History and the Last Man*. In his book, Fukuyama famously predicted the collapse of the Soviet Union and the fall of the Berlin wall. Fukuyama was really talking about the end of an ideological revolution. He claimed that liberal democracy would eventually overcome rival ideologies, including hereditary monarchies, fascism, communism and dictatorships.

I am not predicting the collapse of the National Health Service or the demise of American Health Care, but neither can be sustained in its present form. No amount of tinkering will solve the problems. The future will be determined by the economic reality.

This book is not about the economics of medicine, although that is examined. It is concerned with the radical changes taking place in medicine, as it edges towards an endpoint, the eradication of premature disease. Some of these changes have to do with the advance of science and the technological revolution. But most have to do with the philosophical shift that will be required by patients and doctors to adjust to these changes. The physician is now a mélange of health professionals, part man/woman, part machine.

Fukuyama has been accused of wishful thinking, and labelled a palaeolithic neocon. He has modified his views. But the changes that confront medicine are profound. It is not going to be more of the same.

It is said that schoolchildren celebrate Fukuyama, thinking that if history has ended, algebra can't be far behind. Maybe adults will welcome the end of doctors, thinking lawyers must be next.

SL

---

1. Fukuyama F. *The End of History and The Last Man*. Avon Books: New York, 1993.

About the author

Sidney Lowry began his career as a physicist at Newcastle Royal Victoria Infirmary, where he was involved in calibrating the first Linear Accelerator for cancer therapy. Moving to the City of Dublin Cancer Hospital, he covered the opening of Calder Hall, Sellafield, the world's first nuclear power station, for *The Irish Times*.

He began his medical studies at The University of Virginia in Charlottesville, completing his degree back in Ireland in under four years. Returning to Boston as an Assistant Professor at the New England Medical Center, he pioneered brachytherapy for prostate cancer with Fernando Bloedorn. He also wrote the first joint textbook on radiotherapy and chemotherapy, translated into several languages.

Appointed to the new Chair of Oncology at Queen's University, Belfast, he published widely on cancer and related topics, and held office on a number of international bodies. In one novel report in *The Lancet*, he showed how human body temperature is set at 37°C, the equilibrium point on Isaac Newton's exponential Law of Cooling, a finding he describes as consistent with the music of the primes.

He retired four times, most recently as consultant oncologist and Chairman of the Bermuda Tumour Board. He also held locum posts in Waterford, Wexford and Kilkenny, and acted as advisor on clinical trials to the Irish Medicines Board. Currently serves on the council of the Northern Ireland Medico-Legal Society.

Married with four children, he lives in Co Down. He plays piano, golf, tennis and bridge, in descending order.

Acknowledgements

A sea change is taking place in medicine, and few are talking about it. It involves the changing roles of doctors and, just as significantly, the changing expectations of patients.

This transformation was taking place gradually until recently, then suddenly it gathered pace. This book is an attempt to chronicle the sequence of events, and grapple with the implications. The text began as notes for an essay, until I became aware of the magnitude of the change. One event was significant. It was an oration delivered by Lord Carswell, the former Law Lord, to The Ulster Medical Society in 2003. His talk was entitled, "Consent to medical treatment – Does doctor know best?" My book is not a response to that lecture, and certainly not a rebuttal. But the lecture was a starting point, an incentive; and it prompted me to develop the theme. My thanks to Bob Carswell.

The other incentive came from the thousands of patients I have seen and treated over the years, on both sides of the Atlantic. Sadly many are now deceased. My hope is that some of them may become alive again in these pages.

Many others guided me along the way. Among them I must mention Jim Sharkey, who drew my attention to the decline of compassion in medicine; Jim Dornan, who set me right about the challenges of obstetrics; Sheena Lewis who enlightened me on advances in reprogenetics; Neil Gordon who updated me on changes in pharmaceutical regulations; and Frank Read and Peter Hedstrom who told me the remarkable story of the Barraquer dynasty.

I am especially grateful to Michael Scott for his poem 'Witch's Glove', and the *Irish Medical Journal* for permission to publish it. Special thanks are due to Alison Campbell, Mark Sanderson and the staff at RSM Press for their helpful advice and encouragement.

I drew inspiration from the writings of Marcia Angell and Arnold Relman. Their courageous stand on behalf of integrity in medicine deserves recognition everywhere. And there were others whose influence permeates the book, including Alice Trillin, Barbara Ehrenreich, Sheila Hancock and Lewis Thomas. I am grateful to them all.

Many others were involved, too numerous to mention, or indeed recall, who contributed with ideas and experiences. The book profited enormously from spirited conversations with friends and colleagues.

I thank them all and absolve them from all responsibility for what appears in the text. The views are mine, and mine alone, and were refined by reading and discussion.

Writing a book is a pleasure and a challenge, but occasionally a chore. Putting it all together is a major task. Some I know can put pen to paper and the immediate result is deathless prose. For myself, I take my cue from GBS, who said the rewrite is the thing. I could have taken another year revising endlessly. But there comes a time when one must draw a line, a deadline, and send the manuscript to press. This is difficult when writing about the future – for what is written today may be out of date tomorrow, especially in medical science. Fortunately I have been able to include two startling advances in the text: first, Craig Venter created artificial life out of inert molecules; second, some in the shadows have formed hybrid embryos, half human, half animal. These developments are significant signposts in the rocky path that lies ahead.

Finally I must thank my family, all of whom have been supportive and contributed in different ways. Above all my wife Barbara, who has tolerated my forays at the computer keyboard in the middle of the night, and painstakingly read and corrected the text from cover to cover. All have my enduring love and appreciation.

As the Emperor said to Mozart, "Well, there it is".

SL

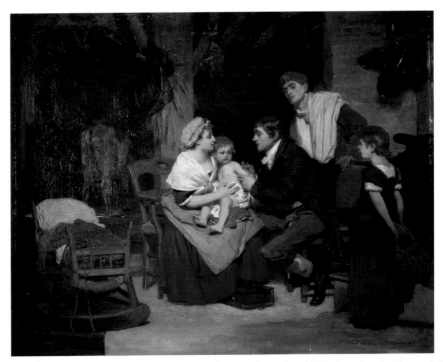

Plate 1 *Edward Jenner vaccinating a boy. Oil painting by E-E Hillemacher, 1884. Reproduced with permission of the Wellcome Library, London.*

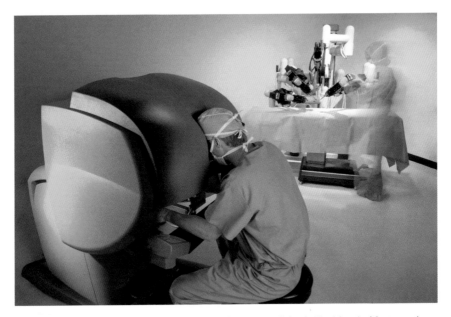

Plate 2 *Robotic surgery: a surgeon is able to command the actions of the da Vinci Surgical System using a master console that has binocular vision of the entire surgical procedure and guides delicate devices through the incisions. Reproduced with permission. © 1999 Intuitive Surgical, Inc.*

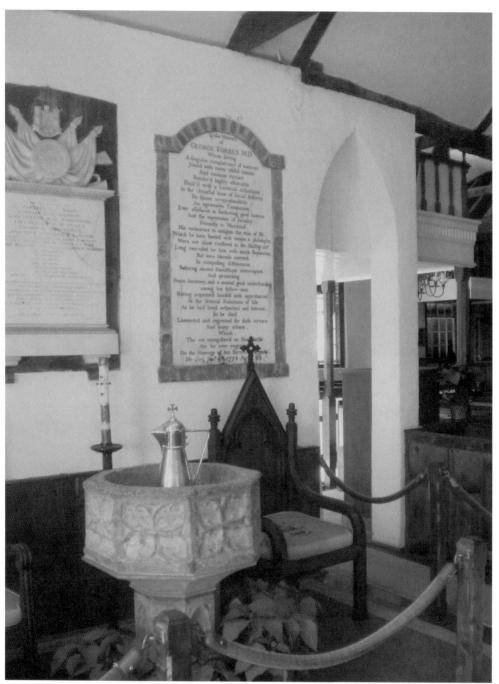

Plate 3 *George Forbes, MD: an 18th century memorial tablet to a revered physician, in St Peter's Church, Bermuda – the oldest continuously used Anglican Church in the Western Hemisphere.*

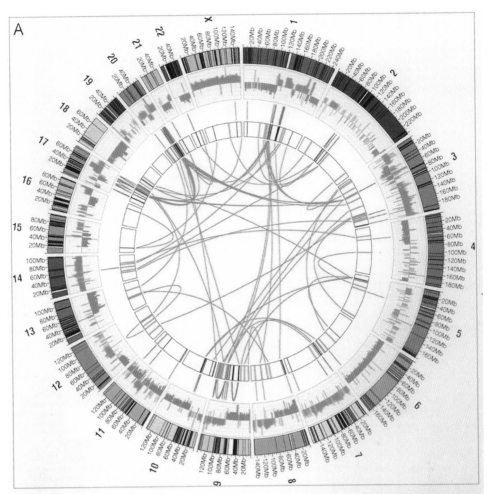

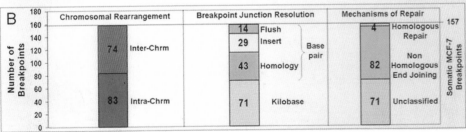

Plate 4 *Chaotic genome. This graphic is a circular visualization of a cancer genome: the outer ring consists of the chromosomes; the middle rings show aberrations, including mutations; and the red lines in the bull's eye denote switches between chromosomes.*[1] *Reproduced with permission of the author and Cold Spring Harbor Laboratory Press.*

Reference
1. Hampton OA, Den Hollander P, Miller CA, Delgado DA et al. A sequence-level map of chromosomal breakpoints in the MCF-7 breast cancer cell line yields insights into the evolution of a cancer genome. *Genome Research* 2009; **19(2)**: 167–77.

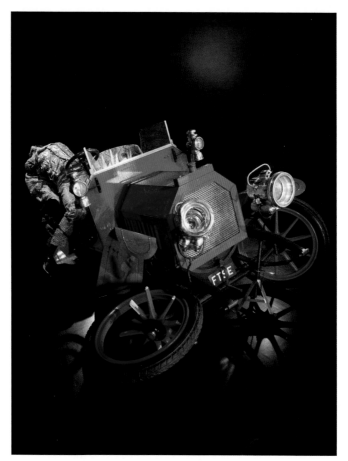

Plate 5 *'Crash Willy' 2009 by Yinka Shonibare. This sculptural dramatization of a headless mannequin astride a car wreck is based on the death of Willy Loman, Arthur Miller's tragic protagonist in* Death of a Salesman, *and also on the earliest photograph of a fatal car crash. This exhibit was the centrepiece of the Royal Academy's Summer Exhibition in London in 2010. Reproduced with permission. Image © the artist and Stephen Friedman Gallery, London. Photograph courtesy of Stephen White.*

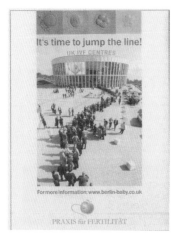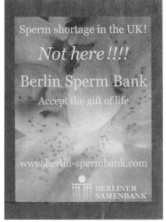

Plate 6 *An advertisement for German IVF treatment, from the in-flight magazine of a popular airline. Reproduced with permission of Berliner Samenbank.*

CHAPTER 1

Preamble

Unfolding the Great Mystery: *In the beginning was the word, and the word was zygote. The zygote was without form and there was darkness in the womb. On the fifth day the zygote begat the blastocyst, and the stem cells went forth to create the embryo. Throughout gestation the fetus basked in an amniotic sea. And it came to pass in the ninth month that the infant was delivered into the light.*

Yet its days were numbered, as foretold in the code encrypted in its genome.

These things, sexual reproduction and death, the beginning and the end, are written in the literature of the ages. They bear witness to the continuity of the human race, and the finality of the individual.

> **Chapter summary**
> • The four phases

Medicine has been involved throughout this process. Not content with its traditional role, medicine has been tampering at both ends of the life cycle, from conception and the zygote to the coffin and beyond.

Meanwhile the healing art has given way to the cold concept of evidence-based medicine. Gradually the physician is being replaced by the machine. Patients no longer want to be examined. They want an MRI. The laying on of hands has been lost. The machine has no feelings, no compassion. This marks the end of clinical medicine as we have known it.

What we may also be witnessing is not just the end of a chapter, but the end of conventional medicine as such: the eventual triumph of science over *premature* disease. Already life expectancy in the West far exceeds the biblical span of threescore years and ten. Although stubborn residual problems remain, progress has been rapid and the outlook is favourable. This is good news.

Yet there is a paradox: The success of medicine has created new phenomena, not all of them benign – overpopulation, increased longevity, frailty and senescence. Coping with these changes is primarily a socio-economic problem, largely beyond the scope and capability of the medical profession.

At the same time, there has been an attitudinal change. Doctors are increasingly challenged – by politicians, by the media, by patients themselves, by the threat of litigation, and even on the fringe by alternative medicine. Doctor no longer knows best.

I propose to show how these changes have come about, and share the crystal gazing with the reader. This story is not about the failure of medicine. It is about the consequences of its success.

The four phases

Advances in health care can be traced from antiquity to the present day. The beginnings of medicine and the first doctors are obscured in a fog of history. Not much happened until relatively recently, then all at once many diseases were brought under control. Most of the progress occurred in the last 150 years. In a short span of time, we have moved from leeches, potions and rituals to epigenetics and nanomedicine.

The first of four phases began in the 19th century. The germ theory was established, and the organisms of many diseases were identified in the laboratory. These ranged from bubonic plague and cholera to syphilis and tuberculosis. Epidemiology, public health and hygiene also played a part in improving survival.

The second phase followed in the 1920s with the discovery of insulin and penicillin. Vaccination against smallpox, poliomyelitis, measles, mumps and rubella (MMR), and influenza brought further improvements.

The third phase involved changes in lifestyle through health education, protection, screening and prevention programmes. The importance of diet, nutrition and exercise, and the dangers of smoking, were emphasized.

A fourth phase is already underway with molecular intervention. All of these advances eradicated many of the causes of premature death, edging life expectancy into the eighties.

Having traced the historical sequence of events, the book then examines health care in Britain and the USA. A common pattern emerges. Most of the budget is spent at the end of life, attempting to extend survival. Problem areas are examined, including malpractice and defensive medicine, the loss of compassion, disease mongering, and a rise of the worried well.

The *End of Medicine* attempts to explain this fundamental – and yet strangely unnoticed – shift in the nature of health care. It involves the changing roles of doctors, and, at least as significantly, the changing expectations of the public.

The 57 subspecialties of medicine and surgery have been struggling to adjust to the new era. A government report in Britain in 2006, on modernizing medical careers, resulted in turmoil among junior doctors. The then Minister of Health was forced to apologize. In 2008, Professor Sir John Tooke led an Independent Review.[1] Among its findings, the authoritative inquiry found no consensus on the future role of the doctor. This conclusion was not surprising, considering the accelerating pace of change. Science is moving ahead so rapidly, it is leaving ethics, morality and law behind.

A closer look at these achievements promises a new era, but it will not be an era in which the doctor holds sway. The future of health care will look very different.

References

1. Catto G, Brown M, Black C et al. The Tooke Report: responses from the profession. *British Journal of Hospital Medicine* 2008; **69**: 68–9.

CHAPTER 2

The legacy of antiquity

Some years ago, Alvin Toffler wrote a book entitled *Future Shock*.[1] In it, he stated that the future was arriving so quickly that we have been unable to adjust fully to the changes. He noted that more scientific advances had occurred in his lifetime than in the whole of previous history. This is certainly true of medicine. Medicine is suffering from a severe case of *Toffler's syndrome*.

Chapter summary
- Anatomy and physiology
- Bloodletting and purgatives
- The barber surgeons

To understand the rapidity of these changes, we need to spend a moment looking at the history of medicine throughout the ages. The story began a long time ago.

Much of ancient medicine was backward, with emphasis on witchcraft, potions and incantations. Even today, witch doctors persist in parts of the developing world, and equally bizarre beliefs continue to be held by some in the developed world.

Nonetheless, early medicine was not entirely primitive. There were many remarkable observations and developments throughout the ages. These date back to Babylonia, Egypt, China, Persia and ancient Greece.

The Kahun Papyrus from Egypt dates from around 1800 BC, and is the oldest surviving medical text.[2] It deals primarily with childbirth and gynaecological conditions. In Pakistan, evidence has been uncovered of teeth having been drilled several thousand years earlier. Chinese medicine is often associated with acupuncture, but the Taoist physicians also made careful observations of the signs and symptoms of many illnesses. The history of Hebrew medicine is documented in the Torah. Many of the Jewish commands and rituals are based on religious belief founded on sound health practice.

The outstanding contribution of ancient Greece to medicine is well known. Hippocrates drafted the Hippocratic Oath, and made perceptive clinical observations along with his pupils. Equally in Rome, Galen pioneered many surgical procedures, including removal of cataracts. Not surprisingly, the Romans continued to develop medicine and surgery up until the fall of the Western Roman Empire in the 5th century.

After the fall, vestiges of European culture survived in the monasteries, such as the island outpost of Skellig Michael, off the coast of southern Ireland. But the church was more concerned with the soul and the sins of the flesh than with the health of the population. Medical practice virtually vanished and the Dark Ages followed.

Fortunately, the bulk of classical knowledge moved east to the Byzantine Empire in Constantinople, but not for long. When the Emperor Justinian disbanded Plato's School of Philosophy in Athens in 529, some of its pupils found refuge in Persia, which had also sheltered the excommunicated Nestorian scholars from Constantinople the previous century. The spread of Islam merged with Byzantine scholarship, and the values of antiquity were thereby preserved and fostered in the Arab world.

The enlightened Abbasid Caliphate in Baghdad, at the end of the 8th century, was followed by many talented names, including translators, alchemists, epidemiologists and clinicians. Ali-Raza was born in 841 near Teheran, but moved to Baghdad. A brilliant physician and thinker, he studied paediatrics, kidney stones, malaria, scabies, hygiene, diet, drugs and epidemiology. Centuries before his time, he denounced quackery and charlatans, and wrote extensively on the doctor/patient relationship.

Shortly after, ibn Sina (Avicenna) was born in Uzbekistan and later moved to Persia. A philosopher, scientist, musician, poet, and physician, he has been called the father of modern medicine. Among many achievements, he introduced the thermometer and proposed quarantine in contagious diseases. Notably, he wrote the *Canon of Medicine*, over one million words, that was to remain the standard textbook in Europe and Asia from the 11th to the 17th century.

Around the same time further west, Abulcasis (936–1013), Islam's greatest surgeon, was born in Andalucía in Moorish Spain. He invented many surgical tools, including the scalpel, forceps, and devices for examining the ear and urethra and removing foreign bodies from the throat. Abulcasis was the first to describe ectopic pregnancy, and he too wrote a 30-volume encyclopaedia of medicine and surgery.

European medicine re-emerged from the Dark Ages with the opening of a medical school in Salerno, Italy in the 11th century. Although there were hiccups along the way, from that time on modern medicine began to take shape.

Anatomy and physiology

Human anatomy had been described in cave drawings from earliest times. A glance at Leonardo da Vinci's drawings in the 15th century reveals the detail that continued to be recorded by many artists, including Rembrandt. The academic study of the human body was subsequently documented in the meticulous drawings of the Flemish anatomist Andreas Vesalius in the 16th century. Vesalius was born in Brussels in 1514 and died 50 years later. His Opus Magnus[3] was entitled *De Humanie Corporis Fabrica*. His studies were later consolidated by the English anatomist Henry Gray. Gray was born in 1827 and tragically died at the age of 34 of smallpox, contracted from his nephew. *Gray's Anatomy* remains the standard anatomical text on both sides of the Atlantic to the present day.

Physiology came to prominence following the work of William Harvey, born in 1578. Harvey was the first to describe the pumping function of the heart and the circulation of the blood. He was born during the golden age of Elizabeth I in England, and was supported by her successors James I and Charles I. Science was moving forward rapidly in England. Harvey died when Isaac Newton was a teenager. Harvey's work was widely accepted in England, but his results were treated with scepticism on the continent.

Bloodletting and purgatives

Although anatomy, physiology and the scientific method moved rapidly forward following the work of Vesalius and Harvey, it is extraordinary that medical practice hardly changed for another 200 years. Some years ago, the Yale physiologist and historian Howard Wilcox Haggard[4] described the ludicrous attempts to treat the dying King Charles II – and this took place during the lifetime of Isaac Newton (see box).

The late Professor Gary Love[5] and others[6] have noted that things were not very different a century later in the USA. George Washington, who was a fit man in his sixties, suffered a foundering after inspecting his farms on horseback in the freezing rain and snow in 1799. The next morning, he awoke with quinsy, laryngitis and pneumonia. A blistering poultice was applied to his neck. He was then required to gargle with a mixture of calomel, vinegar and molasses, and bled five pints of blood. This led to shock and dehydration. Exhausted, he said: 'I thank you for your attentions, but I pray you, take no more trouble about me.' When the doctors retired, his last words were 'Tis well.'

The barber surgeons

The distinction between physicians and surgeons goes back several centuries, and persists today. Although surgical procedures were carried out in ancient cultures, the surgeon was often considered the technician, whereas the physician was the healer and the intellectual. In Britain, surgeons continue to be addressed as Mister and physicians as Doctor. This dates back to the time of the surgical barbers. The continued use of this form of address is a curious case of inverted snobbery that bemuses American doctors.

Originally the surgical barbers consisted of two groups: those who were primarily concerned with cutting hair and shaving, and those who were involved in bloodletting and other surgical procedures. The Royal College of Surgeons of Edinburgh is the oldest surgical society. It has been in continuous existence since 1505, when it was incorporated as a craft guild of the city of Edinburgh. In England, the surgeons and barbers were united by Henry VIII in 1540 as the Worshipful Company of Barbers.

The dying King Charles II

At eight o'clock on Monday 2 February 1685, King Charles II of England was being shaved in his bedroom. With a sudden cry, he fell backward and had a violent convulsion. He became unconscious, rallied once or twice, and after a few days died. Doctor Scarburgh, one of 14 physicians called to treat the stricken king, recorded the efforts made to cure the patient.

As the first step in treatment, the king was bled to the extent of a pint from a vein in the right arm. Next, his shoulder was incised and the area cupped to suck out an additional eight ounces of blood. After this, drugging began. An emetic and purgative were administered, and soon after a second purgative. This was followed by an enema containing antimony, sacred bitters, rock salt, mallow leaves, violets, beet root, camomile flowers, fennel seed, linseed, cinnamon, cardamom seed, saffron, cochineal and aloes. The enema was repeated in two hours and a purgative given. The king's head was shaved and a blister raised on his scalp. A sneezing powder of hellebore root was administered, and also a powder of cowslip flowers to strengthen his brain. The cathartics were repeated at frequent intervals and interspersed with a soothing drink composed of barley water, liquorice and sweet almond. Likewise, white wine, absinthe and anise were given, as also were extracts of thistle leaves, mint, rue and angelica. For external treatment, a plaster of Burgundy pitch and pigeon dung was applied to the king's feet. The bleeding and purging continued, and the following medicaments were added: melon seeds, slippery elm and black cherry water, an extract of flowers of lime, lily of the valley and peony lavender, and dissolved pearls. Still to come were gentian root, nutmeg, quinine and cloves.

The king's condition did not improve; in fact, it grew worse, and in the emergency 40 drops of extract of human skull were administered to allay convulsions. A rallying dose of Raleigh's antidote was forced down the king's throat: the antidote contained an enormous number of herbs and animal extracts. Finally, bezoar stone was given.

'Then alas,' said Scarburgh, 'after an ill-fated night, his serene majesty's strength seemed exhausted to such a degree that the whole assembly of physicians lost all hope and became despondent; still, so as not to appear in failing to do their duty in any detail, they brought into play the most active cordial.' As a sort of grand summary to this pharmaceutical debauch, a mixture of Raleigh's antidote, pearl julep and ammonia was forced down the throat of the dying king.

By the 17th century, the surgeons and barbers began to separate finally, although bloodletting, using either the razor or leeches, persisted for many years. An additional legal perk was granted in England and Scotland at that time – the bodies of a limited number of executed criminals were donated for the purpose of dissection. Three distinguished surgeons in England, Scotland and Ireland pioneered surgery in the early years.

Percival Pott was born in London in 1714. He was the first to describe the splinting of bone fractures. He is best known for his eponyms: Pott's fracture of the ankle and Pott's disease or tuberculosis of the spine. Surgeon Pott also described the hydrocele, the inguinal hernia and fistula-in-ano. Equally important, he recognized an association between soot and chimney sweepers' cancer of the scrotum, a first in epidemiology. Pott was elected a Fellow of the Royal Society.

The second distinguished surgeon was his pupil John Hunter, born in Scotland in 1728. Hunter was the youngest of 10 children, several of whom did not survive infancy. He made many original observations in dentistry, inflammation and gunshot wounds. Notably, he described the lymphatic system and recognized the separation of the fetal and maternal circulations. Hunter was kind to his patients, but could also be irascible. Rather dubiously, he acquired the skeleton of the 7 foot 7 inch Irish giant Charles Byrne and made detailed anatomical observations, which still reside in the Hunterian library of the Royal College of Surgeons. Hunter was also elected to The Royal Society.

The third surgeon of that era was Abraham Colles, born in Ireland in 1773. Colles was a distinguished anatomist and wrote the definitive text on surgical anatomy. He studied many topics, ranging from venereal disease, rampant in Europe, to club foot and vascular surgery. Interestingly, although not correct on detail, he recognized a form of passive immunity in infants born from mothers with syphilis. Colles' fascia of the perineum was named after him. His other eponym is Colles' fracture of the distal radius, an observation far ahead of its time, preceding the discovery of X-rays.

Neither Percival Pott nor John Hunter were awarded knighthoods, although their predecessors the physicians Sir Thomas Browne and Sir Thomas Sydenham were decorated 100 years previously. Colles, who died a few years after Pott and Hunter, and lived on into the 19th century, was offered a baronetcy but, for whatever reason, declined the honour.

Surgery only began to move forward later when its three principal obstacles were overcome. These were pain, bleeding and infection. By the 18th century, the stage was set for the age of diagnosis.

References

1. Toffler A. *Future Shock*. Bantam Books: New York, 1970.
2. Breasted H. *The Edwin Smith Surgical Papyrus*. University of Chicago Press, 1930.
3. Vesalius A. *De Humanie Corporis Fabrica*. Paduan Lectures. 16th century.
4. Haggard HW. *Devils, Drugs and Doctors*. Harper, New York, 1929.
5. Love AGH. Serving two masters. *Ulster Medical Journal* 1989; **58**: 13–28.
6. Silverman WA. The public character of scientific medicine. *Perspectives in Biology and Medicine* 1983; **26**: 343–53.

CHAPTER 3

The age of diagnosis

Long before effective treatments were devised for illnesses, doctors began the task of identifying and describing various diseases. Mostly the conditions and their clinical manifestations were named after the physicians who described them.

Chapter summary

- Scientific advances
- Therapeutic nihilism
- The transition

Literally thousands of eponyms were attached to laboratory tests, clinical symptoms, signs and numerous diseases. Many of these have long since disappeared, but some well-known names survive. These include Parkinson's disease, Hodgkin's disease, Raynaud's phenomenon, Eustachian tube, Cushing's disease, Münchausen syndrome, Colles' fracture and the Heimlich manoeuvre. Curiously, the somewhat clumsy eponym Wolff–Parkinson–White persists to describe an unusual cardiac arrhythmia. Perhaps best known of all is Alzheimer's disease.

It was due to the detailed observations of these physicians and many others that the classification of diseases was founded. Nevertheless, therapeutic nihilism persisted right up until the 20th century. Diseases only began to be controlled by prevention, through discoveries in epidemiology.

Scientific advances

Physics

The impact of physics on medicine has a long history and continues today. Arguably the most important early breakthrough was the development of microscopy by Anton Philips van Leeuwenhoek (1632–1723), born in the Netherlands. Leeuwenhoek did not invent the microscope: the earliest lenses date back to ancient Egypt and Babylon, and the first primitive microscope was made by a Moor in Spain, Abbas Ibn Firnas, a polymath born in Rondo in the 9th century. Leeuwenhoek, however, was the first to develop the modern science of microbiology. He made over 500 microscopes, which he used to identify bacteria and microorganisms. He laid the foundations for the work of Pasteur and others to follow.

Gabriel Fahrenheit devised a temperature scale in 1724 using a mercury thermometer. He based his scale on the range between the freezing point of salt water and human body temperature. This enabled biologists and others to use units that for the most part did not involve negative numbers. It also allowed for finer temperature increments, not possible on the Celsius scale. It was helpful in early studies, but is now mainly of historical and academic interest; curiously, it survives in the USA.

Benjamin Franklin is credited with inventing the first pair of bifocal spectacles in 1760. Although hardly a dramatic discovery, it was and remains a useful visual aid for the elderly.

The invention of the stethoscope was not in the same category as the discovery of X-rays, but it was nonetheless an important milestone in the clinical examination of patients. The stethoscope was invented by Rene Laennec, a physician in France in 1816. Laennec's invention was based on the science of acoustics. Auscultation has been central to the physical examination of patients ever since. It complements percussion, again based on the physics of sound, which was pioneered by the Austrian physician Leopold Auenbrugger in 1761.

Hermann von Helmholtz was both a physicist and a physician. He studied the science of optics in Germany, and in 1851 invented the ophthalmoscope, an essential tool for the clinical examination of the retina.

Although Michael Faraday (1791–1867) does not feature in the history of medicine, his early work following the discovery of electricity made an enormous impact on the 19th century, including the medical sciences. Faraday is credited with many outstanding achievements beyond his work on electromagnetism, including studies on industrial pollution and the origin of nanoscience. Although a Fellow of the Royal Society, he twice refused to become its President. He also declined a knighthood.

Among the many names that led to advances in classical physics were William Crookes and JJ Thompson. Crookes, born in London in 1832, was both a chemist and a physicist. He investigated the conduction of electricity in gases and invented the Crookes vacuum tube. Thomson, born in Manchester in 1856 of Scottish descent, then used a Crookes tube to pursue conduction studies leading to the discovery of electrons, a revelation for which he won the Nobel Prize. But it was not until the following century that the study of conduction by electrons in the gaseous state moved to the solid state of semiconductors; a discovery that was to transform medicine, and indeed almost every aspect of the modern world (see e-health later).

The German physicist Wilhelm Conrad Roentgen (1845–1923) deserves a special place in the history of medicine. His discovery of X-rays ranks alongside the work of Pasteur. It marked the beginning of diagnostic radiology and imaging. In some ways, his discovery also anticipated the current move away from the clinical examination of patients, to diagnosis by machine. The discovery also led to the foundation of therapeutic radiology or radiation oncology, a cornerstone of cancer treatment. Roentgen was awarded the first Nobel Prize in physics in 1901.

Roentgen's discovery paralleled the work of Marie Curie (1867–1934). Marie Sklodowska from Poland married Pierre Curie from France and spent much of her life in Paris. She extended the work of Henri Becquerel, who discovered that uranium salts emitted radiation that resembled X-rays (1896). Marie Curie discovered radium, coined the term 'radioactivity' and isolated radioactive isotopes. As with Roentgen, her work predicted the specialty of nuclear medicine, and had applications in both cancer therapy and radio diagnosis. She was awarded two Nobel Prizes.

The discovery of the electrocardiograph in The Netherlands in 1903 was the work of the physicist and physician Willem Einthoven. It was already known that the beating heart produced electrical impulses. But these could only be measured by placing electrodes directly on the heart. Einthoven developed the string galvanometer, a highly sensitive instrument that allowed accurate readings to be taken on the chest wall, despite the insulation of the rib cage and soft tissues. He too was awarded a Nobel Prize.

Physicians in the 17th century knew of the existence of blood pressure in animals, but had no means of measuring it. The Austrian physician Samuel Siegfried Karl Ritter von Basch (1837–1905) is usually credited with inventing the sphygmomanometer. Others were involved in its development, including Harvey Cushing in Baltimore in 1901. The early physicians used their fingers to palpate the pulse of arterial blood flow, but it was left to the Russian surgeon Nicolai Korotkov in 1905 to combine the use of the stethoscope to listen to the sounds of blood flow through the brachial artery. Again, today hypertension can be detected by machine without the need of a physician.

Microbiology

Interestingly, the first major advance in microbiology involved not a bacterium, but a virus, variola, the cause of smallpox. There is evidence that the practice of inoculating groups of people with small amounts of virus existed in ancient China, and later in America and parts of Europe. The practice was potentially dangerous, not widespread and not well documented. Edward Jenner FRS (1749–1823) is given the credit for introducing a much safer procedure (see Colour Plate 1). Jenner was an English GP and surgeon who trained under John Hunter. He noted that milkmaids infected with cowpox, a related virus, did not develop smallpox. He decided to inoculate an 8-year-old boy, James Phipps, with cowpox, and subsequently performed the same procedure on 23 other people. Most did well, and although a few later developed smallpox, it was much less virulent. Today, his experiment would be considered irresponsible and unethical. Jenner must have been convinced he was right. He was probably unaware that several others had also tested cowpox vaccination, since their work was not widely known. Mass vaccination against smallpox was eventually introduced worldwide, and ultimately led to the eradication of the disease. Jenner was a meticulous scientist. He was interested in nature, and had studied the life cycle of the cuckoo and the migration of birds.[1]

Garcia de Orta, a Portuguese physician, was the first European to describe cholera, in Goa around 1560. But it was not until 1832, when the English physician

John Snow mapped out the incidence of cholera in London, that the disease was controlled. Snow identified a cluster of cases around a single contaminated well, dug three feet from a cesspit in Soho. Convinced that cholera was a waterborne disease, Snow persuaded the council to remove the pump handle in Broad Street and the disease diminished. Snow was sceptical of the miasma theory, which claimed that diseases were caused by pollution or bad air. The government accepted his findings but rejected his theory, having a distaste for the concept of oral–faecal transmission. Snow also pioneered anaesthesia, devising dosimetry for chloroform and ether. He anaesthetized Queen Victoria during the birth of two of her children. In a recent medical poll, he was voted to be one of the greatest physicians of all time. Sadly, he died when he was only 45 years old.

Ignaz Semmelweiss in Vienna in 1847 realized that puerperal sepsis, a cause of maternal death, was contagious and transmitted by doctors. He recommended that obstetricians wash their hands before delivering infants, and dramatically reduced the maternal death rate. However, many still rejected the germ theory of disease, claiming that diseases were due to an imbalance of humours. Semmelweiss spent years trying to convince colleagues and others, but in vain. He became increasingly angry and tragically died in an asylum aged 47 years. Coincidentally, Oliver Wendell Holmes in America reached similar conclusions in a paper published in 1843 entitled 'The contagiousness of puerperal fever'.

In the year of Semmelweiss's death (1865), Joseph Lister, an English surgeon working in Scotland, championed the ideas of Holmes and Semmelweiss and introduced antisepsis to surgery. Scrubbing up has been central to surgery ever since. Lister was elevated to a peerage and became President of The Royal Society.

Twenty years later, in 1885, Louis Pasteur made medical history in Paris, finally confirming the germ theory, and linking microorganisms with disease. Pasteur's legendary work included the introduction of attenuated vaccines, especially for rabies. Like his predecessor Edward Jenner, Pasteur vaccinated a young boy who had been bitten by a rabid dog. Fortunately, it was a great success, for, unlike Jenner, Pasteur was not a medical physician, and failure could have led to litigation!

Following on from Pasteur's work, Robert Koch (1843–1910), a German physician and bacteriologist, isolated the bacteria responsible for anthrax, tuberculosis and cholera, all within the space of 6 years. Then, in 1894, the French/Swiss physician Alexandre Yersin from the Pasteur Institute, working in Hong Kong, isolated *Yersinia pestis*, the organism responsible for the Black Death or bubonic plague, confirming that it was transmitted by fleas from infected rats.

Around the same time, Ronald Ross, an 'army brat' born in India, noted that mosquitoes were breeding in a water tub beneath his bedroom window. He overturned the tub, and suggested to the adjutant that life would be more pleasant if there was no standing water for the parasites to breed in. But his suggestion was treated with derision. Ross went on to prove the role of mosquitoes in transmitting malaria and was honoured with a knighthood. In the Americas, Carlos Finlay in Cuba and Walter Reed in the US army likewise showed that the yellow fever virus was also transmitted by mosquitoes.

These successes were quickly followed by isolation of the organisms responsible for typhoid fever, diphtheria, leprosy, syphilis, meningitis, and many other diseases. The 19th century ended in a medical whirlwind of discoveries.[2] The age of therapy, however, was still around the corner.

Therapeutic nihilism

Sir William Osler (1849–1919), the distinguished Canadian physician, bridged the gap between the 19th and 20th centuries. Osler was a polymath: a clinician, pathologist, essayist, humourist and historian. He held posts at McGill in Montreal, Johns Hopkins in Baltimore, and Oxford. He has been called the Father of Modern Medicine. Osler pioneered bedside teaching for medical students. His textbook *The Principles and Practice of Medicine* was the classic text for decades, right up to the end of the 20th century.

Yet Osler lived in the era of therapeutic nihilism. The academic challenge for physicians was to make accurate diagnoses, not to treat patients. One of the early radiation therapists, the late Dr Arnold Lyons, told me that even up until the 1930s, he had been 'ribbed' by one of his senior colleagues in London, who quipped: 'You don't actually treat patients, old boy, do you?' And as a medical student myself, I recall how we would stand around the bedside, being quizzed on the physical signs and symptoms of a particular patient. And when the diagnosis was made, we would move quickly on to the next bedside.

The transition

Following the establishment of the germ theory in the 19th century, medicine moved forward rapidly. The transition to the therapeutic age began with the discovery of insulin by Banting and Best in Canada in 1921. The pace of research then quickened, and in 1928 Alexander Fleming discovered penicillin. The therapeutic age was underway. Vaccination, prevention, mass radiography and lifestyle changes quickly followed. Public health improved dramatically. Today life expectancy in the West far exceeds the biblical threescore years and ten. The future of health care has taken a new direction.

References

1. Durant W, Durant A. *The Story of Civilisation, Volumes I–X*. Simon and Schuster: New York, 1954–1967.
2. Bynum WF. *Science and the Practice of Medicine in the 19th Century*. Cambridge University Press, 1994.

CHAPTER 4

The National Disease Service

Although the health care systems of Britain and the USA are very different, they share two common features. Costs are spiralling out of control in both jurisdictions. And most of the budget in each country is spent at the end of life, trying to prolong survival. The reasons for this are discussed separately.

Chapter summary
- The NHS
- NICE
- Dental decay
- A safety net

The NHS

The National Health Service (NHS) in Britain might more accurately be described as the National Disease Service. The emphasis has always been on treatment rather than prevention. Yet the foundation of the NHS marked the beginning of a revolution in health care. The late Donald Soper – the Reverend Lord Soper, the only Methodist clergyman to be elevated to a peerage* for his lifelong commitment to socialism – described the NHS as 'the greatest experiment in practical Christianity in his lifetime'. Soper knew what he was talking about. He knew what it was like in the old days.[1,2] And who are we to argue?

The NHS was ushered in with the welfare state in 1946 and was enacted on 5 July 1948. The father of the Act was Aneurin (Nye) Bevan. He stated 'The collective principle asserts that no society can legitimately call itself civilised if a sick person is denied medical aid because of lack of means.' He added, 'A free health service is pure socialism and is opposed to the hedonism of a capitalist society.'

Churchill called him 'a squalid nuisance'. But Bevan fought the medical profession and the British Medical Association. Finally he brokered a deal with some minor concessions to the consultants. In the end he said that he 'stuffed their mouths with gold!'

One retired family physician,[3] Dr John Marks, said that before the NHS no one realized how much unknown sickness existed in the community. Many

---

* Soper had a keen sense of humour. When he entered the upper chamber, he was surprised at the standard of debate. He said it was living proof of life after death.

could not afford to go to the doctor. The new health service was followed by an unprecedented rush to the GP, with problems people had been putting off for years.[4]

But the dream has faded. What has happened? The short answer is that we can no longer afford it. The idea of free medicine from the cradle to the grave was a noble concept. Originally it included everything for everyone: free prescriptions for all, free dental care, even free reading glasses. In 1948, it was envisaged that the costs of the NHS would go down as health care improved. The opposite has happened, and today costs continue to rise.

Take the super scanner that the Royal Bank of Scotland recently donated to Edinburgh, on condition the bank employees have priority use. It cost £250 million to develop. Critics say it will lead to a two-tier health service. Others claim we already have that with the expansion of private medicine.

But in spite of the problems, no British government would try to turn the clock back. At the outset, Churchill set up a committee to examine the effectiveness of the tax-based system. The committee concluded that the NHS was very effective, and, if anything, needed more money. The Conservatives were furious, but the report ended any attempt to reverse the system.

More recently, after losing three successive elections to Labour, the Conservatives have embraced the system, and are now committed to increased health care funding. Interestingly when the NHS was set up, there were 480,000 hospital beds. Today there are fewer than half that number, despite more people being treated.

Health care is the world's biggest industry, worth in excess of several billion pounds. The NHS is the world's largest employer after Indian Rail, the Chinese Army and Wal-Mart. Think tanks such as the King's Fund, politicians and economists have struggled to analyse the budget, with talk of wastage, efficiency savings, revenue consequences and so on. There are many elements to the financial problems. Increased longevity obviously contributes. So also do patient expectations. There is an increased demand for new investigations, and a clamour for 'wonder drugs'. And there is the spectre of litigation.

In tackling these problems, various governments have mounted a series of reviews, ranging from the 'Patient's Charter', devised by the then British Prime Minister John Major, to the Darzi Review of the subsequent Labour government. Even the new coalition government in 2010 is planning another review. Andrew Lansley, the coalition health secretary, has announced the biggest shake up in the NHS since its foundation in 1948. No wonder doctors and nurses are said to be suffering from 'change fatigue'.

The Labour plan of 2008 was prepared by Lord Darzi, a surgeon. It had some merit. Darzi was appointed as one of the GOATS ('government of all talents'), and presented *The Next Stage Review on the Future of the NHS*.[5] Among his proposals, patients were to be asked for their opinions, and doctors and hospitals rewarded on quality of care.[6] Everyone will produce annual quality reports. But measuring a doctor's skill is difficult, even for doctors. If you want to know how good a surgeon is, you don't ask any doctor, you ask the anaesthesiologist. How much more difficult must it be for a member of the public?

Patients need to trust their doctor and have faith in his or her ability. They like a doctor who has a pleasant, friendly, sympathetic personality – someone who has time to listen to their complaints and respond. This is difficult when there are dozens of patients sitting outside in the waiting room. Again, patients like tests to confirm the diagnosis, and prescriptions for their medication, both of which cost time and money. Measuring all these things requires another layer of bureaucracy to mark, reward or penalize. This doesn't mean it is not worth doing – it would be helpful to know these things. It is just very difficult in practice and it is difficult to get reliable data.

Darzi's slogan was 'localize where possible and centralize where necessary'. Many of his ideas were promising, but some met with opposition from the medical profession. He did not take kindly to the criticism. Government advisors alleged that some doctors were 'laggards', mostly interested in protecting their 'professional boundaries'. A former Health Secretary, Patricia Hewitt, blamed the doctors for the financial trouble. She claimed that there was clinical resistance to change.[7]

Lansley plans to tackle the doctors head on.[8] 'This government has no fear of the unions. What can the BMA do? They could threaten to resign en masse from the NHS, but in the current climate do you think there would be much sympathy for whingeing GPs? On £100,000 a year I don't think so' said one source, 'They may have to get used to doing more for less.' The Minister clearly believes in the 'Golden Rule': *The man who has the gold makes the rules.* But there are doubts about whether Lansley's plans will work. The think tank Civitas has warned against further restructuring, saying the evidence for some of the changes is weak.

Eventually, however, politicians and the public are going to have to come to terms with the reality of the economics. They already have in the USA, where a debate raged about the costs of the Obama proposals for health care reform (see Chapter 5).

In the UK, an analysis by the Institute for Fiscal Studies and the King's Fund in 2009 stated that political pledges to protect further NHS spending will force either tax increases or cuts in budgets.[9] The report concludes that the NHS must prepare for the impending 'financial freeze'. Health costs have grown to more than 9% of gross domestic product (GDP), and about one-fifth of public spending. Something has to give to avoid bankruptcy.

Michael Macdonnell, Director of the 10 Partnership that advised Tony Blair, notes that GPs are gatekeepers to expensive hospital services.[10] 'Every time a referral letter is signed, a bill is created for the NHS.' He believes that 'if the care that follows those letters can be provided by the GP himself, *or by nurses and others*, then money can be saved.' Macdonnell adds that 'strong incentives to keep people healthy and away from the NHS, should in turn impel GPs to encourage people to take part in public health initiatives.' As we shall see later, this has been tried before with limited success. Meanwhile the political manoeuvre may mean that GPs will take the blame for rationing, not the government.

There is an added difficulty that is compounding the problem. It is claimed that patient safety is being put at risk by overworked NHS staff, trying to make the system work.[11] One survey indicated that there were 4000 'avoidable' errors made in the UK in 2008, with more than half of the blunders (2221) considered serious, resulting in injuries and deaths. They included operating on the wrong patient, or the wrong part of the body, the wrong diagnosis and wrong prescriptions.

The problem of overworked doctors led to the introduction of a European Directive, implementing a 48-hour working week for junior doctors. A 48-hour working week is hardly an easy week, yet there were urgent calls from senior doctors for the government to repeal the legislation. The consultants claimed that longer working hours were often necessary so that 'the patients of today and tomorrow get the first class care they deserve'. In my view, a return to overworked juniors deprived of sleep is no solution, especially if it involves another 4000 avoidable errors.

NICE

The rising cost of the health service in England has meant that rationing in some form is inevitable. The National Institute for Health and Clinical Excellence (NICE) was set up for this purpose. Its website states that it is an independent organization responsible for providing national guidance on the promotion of good health and the prevention and treatment of ill health. NICE gives guidance in three areas:

1. Public health
2. Health technologies
3. Clinical practice

Although this watchdog is concerned with clinical excellence, it has been accused of speaking with a 'forked tongue'. Its main task is to consider whether drugs are cost-effective: not whether they are of value, but whether they are value for money.

Lord Kelvin would have liked it, for it puts numbers on it. The cost per life-year saved must be below a threshold of £30,000. The formula used is quite complex. It involves calculating a QALY (quality-adjusted life year). One QALY equals one year of perfect health, or two years of 50% perfect health, or four years of 25% perfect health. All this implies putting numbers on imperfect health, hardly an exact science. If the cost per QALY is under £20,000, the treatment is considered cost-effective and is approved. If it is over that amount but under £30,000, NICE will only approve it in special circumstances. Above that sum, it is only considered in exceptional cases.

The whole system has been widely criticized and is under scrutiny. In reality, it is a form of rationing and may yet be revised or even scrapped. Professor John Harris of the Bioethics Department at Manchester University has likened the system to tossing a coin.[12] In a statement, a spokesperson for NICE said 'We do routinely review our methods for evaluating new treatments and have, with the Department of Health, commissioned research looking at theoretical quality-adjusted life year calculations. This ongoing research is being explored along with a range of issues around cost-effectiveness.'

At the time of writing, when a drug has not been approved by NICE, patients under NHS care are not allowed to top up their treatments privately. This is manifestly absurd and cannot be sustained. At the same time, some of the claims made for new medications are dubious and deserve close inspection (see later).

As a result of widespread criticism, NICE has been constantly revising its recommendations. An NHS select committee subsequently admitted that a two-tier health service was the only realistic way forward, and that top-up drugs should be approved.[13]

Apart from its role in examining the use of new medicines, NICE has also been looking at family practice and prevention. It has proposed that some parts of the arrangement whereby doctors are rewarded both for assessing and for achieving targets should be scrapped – not doing away with targets, but replacing them with new targets. These new targets included lowering the blood pressure in diabetic patients, regular checks for patients with Down syndrome and monitoring patients with epilepsy. The proposed changes to the performance-related pay scheme were the first independent review of targets and bonuses, which account for one-third of GPs' pay.

NICE has also been accused of standing in the way of innovation.[14] It commissioned Professor Sir Ian Kennedy, Emeritus Professor of Health Law, Ethics and Policy at University College, London, to examine the problem. Kennedy found that NICE was in effect a fourth hurdle that stood in the way of innovation. There were already three hurdles to pass before a pharmacological product could be licensed. He noted the clash between the two philosophies: the tension of 'UK Plc needing a vibrant, effective, pharmacological industry for the sake of the economy, and NICE not part of that economic philosophy, but rather a mechanism to allocate scarce resources'. It remains to be seen whether Kennedy's recommendations can reduce the tension.

Interestingly, a clearer idea of the precise role of NICE only emerged after it responded to severe criticism in the furious debate over US health care. Commenting on the US reports about NICE, Sir Andrew Dillon, Chief Executive of NICE, said, 'Comparing health systems is a good way of informing debates about how to get the best for patients. But comparisons need to be accurate and factual. So it's disappointing to read comments about NICE which are untrue or misinformed.' He added, 'The basis of NICE's system of appraising drugs and other treatments is simple: Something will be recommended for use by the NHS, if the benefits for patients are worth what the NHS is being asked to pay. Most new treatments, including some very expensive ones, are worth what the NHS is being asked to pay, which is why we recommend them, for those patients who can really benefit. Some are not, and so we do not encourage the NHS to spend money on them, which could be better used for other things. We don't put a limit on the amount the NHS can spend on an individual patient. But money for the NHS is not limitless. NICE is a force for change and improvement in the NHS, so let's keep the debate about what we do focussed on the facts.'

The fact is that there is a limited pot of money and a degree of rationing in the health service is inevitable. When Andrew Lansley, the Tory Shadow Health Secretary, was in opposition in April 2010, he accused the Labour government of broken promises, denying thousands of cancer patients life-extending drugs. Dillon was quick to respond and said the criticisms of NICE were unfounded. One month later, the conservatives were elected to power, and Lansley was appointed the new Health Secretary. Within hours, it was clear that severe financial restraint was inevitable, and one of the first areas to face cuts would be the NHS.

Americans are sceptical about having a government committee deciding which medical treatments work better than others, but health policy experts say it could help keep down the rising costs. Uwe Reinhardt, a health economist at Princeton University, says, 'The idea that every American has the right to everything imaginable, whether it works or not, is just tragic.' He adds, 'Ultimately that leads to what we have had, where health spending grows 2.5 percentage points faster than the rest of the GDP. For the last 40 years we have had this.' He says that if we continue on this path, in 2050 we will be spending 40% of the GDP on health care.

Dental decay

Dental care is bottom of the NHS league table. Less than two-thirds of children, and less than half of all adults, are registered with a dentist. A government health committee reported in 2009 that the reforms introduced only three years previously had failed to meet their objectives.[15] Dentists were extracting teeth rather than doing complex repair work such as crowns and bridges.[16]

The previous reforms meant that hundreds of dentists opted out of the NHS. One million fewer patients were being treated. Moreover, the contract provided perverse incentives to carry out profitable treatments that were unnecessary. There were also disturbing reports of patients extracting their own teeth because they could not find an NHS dentist. An opposition spokesman in the Liberal Democrat Party, Norman Lamb, said 'The near destruction of NHS dentistry will be one of Labour's most shameful legacies.'

The independent review recommended a return to the old system of rewarding dentists for registering new patients for life. The British Dental Association said the new approach should mean a move away from the 'target-driven arrangements'. The proposals included a three-year guarantee, to stop dentists being paid more to salvage earlier shoddy work.

The proposals also included payments for preventative care and dental hygiene. Interestingly, because of the general improvement in dental hygiene in Britain over the years, many older people in care homes have retained some of their teeth. Unfortunately, however, according to the charity Help the Aged, these senior citizens are now mostly unable to find a dentist. This contrasts with 50 years ago, when half the population had lost all their teeth by the age of 40. Nonetheless, the situation in Scotland has hardly improved. A government report in 2010 found that more than one-third of women over 55, and one-quarter of men, had lost all their teeth.

Someone once said that no one ever died from bad teeth. That is not strictly true. Poor oral hygiene can lead to subacute bacterial endocarditis, and even oral cancer in rare cases. And a report in 2010 states that people who brush their teeth twice daily have a significantly lower rate of heart disease. Even so, the relatively low mortality from dental disease probably accounts for its low priority in the health service.

As for the USA, it was reported in *The Times* of London that Americans could recognize British people from 100 yards by the poor quality of their teeth. Catherine Mayer in *Time* magazine, described the British as a 'snaggletoothed island race'. That may be so, but the comparison is not helpful. Health care in the USA ranges from the very best to the worst (ask Hillary Clinton). I recall our teenage babysitter in New England, who had all her teeth extracted to avoid facing future dental bills. More recently, at the Obama Health Care summit (February 2010), Representative Louise Slaughter, the Democratic congresswoman for New York's 28th District, said she had a constituent whose sister died. 'This poor woman had no dentures. She wore her dead sister's teeth, which were uncomfortable and did not fit. You even believe that in America, that's where we would be?' (see Chapter 5).

Yet at the research level, scientific advances are moving rapidly. A 'plasma jet' that eradicates tooth decay without fillings has been developed in Germany. The device ejects a beam of ionized oxygen atoms into cavities, destroying bacteria. It may soon replace the dentist's drill.

The present book is about the last doctor, not the last dentist. Nevertheless, the possibility of some dentists becoming redundant, because of better dental hygiene, remains an ambivalent goal for the profession.

A safety net

My own view is that the best that the NHS can do today is provide a safety net. And if we accept that definition, it does a fairly good job. The NHS, with all its flaws, remains the goal. But it has to be set within the economic constraints.

First, the government has to stop reacting to special interest groups. The health service should provide basic cover for life-threatening conditions. Anything beyond that must depend on what is left in the kitty. If you want more, you may have to pay for it. Otherwise it is difficult to see how costs can be reduced, even though this entails a two-tier service. Rationing is inevitable.

Second, the money must be spent on the front line. Salaries account for a major part of the expense. In the 10 years from 1998 to 2008, the number of nurses in the NHS grew by 24%. The number of doctors grew by 38%. These figures are effectively lower, for they include women working in a part-time capacity.

In contrast, the number of managers in administration grew by 58%. Only the administrators can reduce the number of bureaucrats in the system. But they are not going to self-destruct. Rather, they may increase to ensure their own survival.

Previous governments set targets. The only target that has not been set is reducing the bureaucratic load. I would commend Warren Buffett's financial dictum. There are two rules:

Rule One: Don't waste money.
Rule Two: Don't forget Rule One.

References

1. Castle T. NHS marks 60th birthday. *Reuters*, 5 July 2008.
2. Triggle N. The NHS – an easy birth. *BBC News*, 25 June 2008.

3. Elliott J. Devoted to the NHS for 60 years. *BBC News*, 2 July 2008.
4. Elliott J. I told Beveridge the NHS was too hurried. *BBC News*, 30 June, 2008.
5. Profile: 'Robo Doc' scrubs up for radical surgery on ailing NHS. *The Sunday Times*, 29 June 2008.
6. Leading Article. World class health costs. *The Times*, 1 July 2008.
7. Kite M, Marsh B. It is the doctors' fault the NHS is in financial trouble, says Hewitt. *The Sunday Telegraph*, 12 March 2006.
8. Ramash R. NHS plan puts the government on collision course with unions and doctors. *The Guardian*, 9 July 2010.
9. NHS spending will force tax hike. *Press Association*, 2 July 2009.
10. Macdonnell M. GPs must do more than manage illness. *The Sunday Times*, 27 June 2010.
11. Overworking blamed for NHS errors. *The Guardian*, April 2009.
12. Smith R. NICE's decisions worse than tossing a coin, says professor. *The Daily Telegraph*, 24 October 2008.
13. Top-up drugs backed. *The Times*, 13 May 2009.
14. Campbell D. Tory cancer claims mislead, says drug body. *The Guardian*, 10 April 2010.
15. Hope J. Labour reverses its dentists' revolution. *Daily Mail*, 23 January 2009.
16. Hawkes N. NHS fails to cure rotten dentistry. *The Times*, 2 July 2008.

CHAPTER 5

Health care in the USA

Health care in the USA cannot easily be compressed into a single chapter. The subject is beyond the scope of this book. Nor can it be omitted, because of its significance in shaping the future of medicine. There are several obvious features.

First, there is the size of the land mass. The USA is not just a country, it is a continent. Many tasks are devolved to individual states. Several of these states are larger than some European countries. Coordinating all this activity across a continent is a massive task. Forging radical change in such circumstances is not easy. There is so much inertia in the system.

Second, the USA was founded by pioneers. Much of the pioneering spirit persists, preserving the freedom and rights of the individual, including the right to reject socialism. Compassion was not a common feature on the frontier. Even today, America is not a country for old men, unless you are financially secure.

Third, within this vast arena there is also a healthy vein of self-criticism. A *Time* magazine contributor once wrote that 'In America if a thing is worth doing, it is worth overdoing.' Latterly the most vociferous American health critic has been Michael Moore, the movie director and activist. His movie *Sicko* portrays the health care scene with a mixture of humour and pathos.

All of these factors impact on health care. It is probably true to say that the USA has the best and the worst of modern medicine. At the top end, the treatment of disease sets a gold standard. If anything, it is overdone, for instance with the aggressive treatment of prostate cancer or the television barrage promoting pharmaceutical products.

Chapter summary

- Health care spending
- Health insurance
- Prescription drug costs
- Health care performance
- Innovation
- Clinton's health plan
- The Obama factor
- Health philosophy
- Doctor substitutes
- The futile pursuit
- Driving up the costs of care
- The historic overhaul
- Too far, or not far enough

At the lower end, 46 million Americans had no health insurance until recently. This has changed, but the extent of the change has yet to be assessed. Alistair Cooke famously remarked that America was founded on three things: compromise, compromise and compromise.

Health care spending

The USA spends more per capita on health care than any other country. Yet it is well down the league table for life expectancy in the Western World. Moreover, infant mortality is higher than in most other developed countries. These statistics have been challenged, but are mostly due to the good results at the upper end of the spectrum being offset by the poor findings at the lower end.

A study in 1996 found that 1% of the population accounted for one-quarter of spending on health care, and 5% for over half of all spending. Of total spending, 31% goes on hospital care, 21% on doctors' fees, 10% on pharmaceuticals, and the balance on other services and administrative costs.

There have been hundreds of insurance companies in the USA involved in health care. This has added to administrative costs. One study found that 30% of the health budget went on administration, twice that of Canada's single-payer system.

Health insurance

About 85% of Americans are covered by some form of health insurance (albeit limited in many cases), mostly provided by employers, with one-quarter coming from government programmes. For many years, the remaining 15% were uninsured. This amounted to 45 million people uninsured.

The government programmes include Medicare, Medicaid, The Children's Health Insurance Program and the Veterans Administration.

Medicare was enacted in 1965. It provides health insurance for people over 65 years old who have been continuously resident in the country for five years. It covers hospital insurance, medical insurance and prescription charges. But there are limitations and deductions, and many patients have to supplement their coverage from other means.

Medicaid was introduced to cover low-income people. Unfortunately, some physicians refuse to accept Medicaid patients, because of low re-imbursement and administrative costs.

The USA has been involved in many foreign conflicts over the years, and ex-service men and women are eligible for care under the Veterans Administration programme. There are restrictions on the amount of support, depending on whether the illness is a service-related disability, and co-payments may be involved.

I worked in both a Veterans Administration hospital and in a private capacity in the USA and can testify that, although the system is heavily criticized, in my experience patients are well treated in both the private and public spheres, regardless of their financial status. That is not to deny that many, including those who were insured, were often financially crippled by the costs of illness. As for the uninsured, they sometimes had to escape into bankruptcy. Indeed, exorbitant medical expenses were cited by half of all those filing for bankruptcy in 2001.

Most health care costs involve the retired community. About half of acute hospital spending occurs during the last two years of life. Medicare remains the main source of cover for these older people, but expenditure has been soaring over the years. One estimate found costs doubling every four years. Predictions suggest that the future is unsustainable, and that the trust will become insolvent in 10 years. There are many reasons for this, but it is mostly because the ratio of younger workers who pay taxes to older retirees receiving services is falling. This ratio is expected to drop even further, as the 'baby boom' generation retires in the coming years. Other factors include the increased costs of new technology and the flood of new drugs onto the market. More worrying is the spectre of waste and even fraud.

Prescription drug costs

As in most countries, the cost of prescription medicine has spiralled in recent years. The USA spends more per capita on pharmaceutical products than any other country, although drug expenditure represents a slightly smaller percentage of overall health care costs compared with other jurisdictions.

Many countries with a single-payer system, and bulk purchasing power, have been able to negotiate lower prices with pharmaceutical companies. However, the Republican Party in the US Congress passed a law in 2005, signed by George W Bush, forbidding Medicare to negotiate drug prices. This infuriated opposition politicians, who claimed that it simply allows drug companies to profiteer off Medicare, which is already in serious financial difficulty. Inevitably, some of this additional cost is passed on to patients who, finding some products not covered by insurance, have to pay for these out of pocket.

Health care performance

As the USA spends the highest amount per capita on health care, one may ask whether the country is getting value for money. The common performance indicators for outcome are survival rate and life expectancy. One report indicated that the 5-year survival rates for many types of cancer in America were the highest in the world. This is often attributed to early diagnosis. The finding, however, has to be interpreted with caution, and adjusted for epidemiological lead-time bias (see later). Patients may appear to survive longer because of the earlier countdown. It is a self-fulfilling prophecy. The earlier you are diagnosed, the longer you will live, *from the time of diagnosis*. Such patients certainly live longer *with the knowledge* they have had cancer.

Moreover, there has been a trend to inflate the grade of malignancy, because of the fear of litigation. Thus, many occult (in situ) cancers of the prostate and breast are included that would never have been life threatening. Indeed one report, in *The Sunday Times* in 2008, noted that some breast cancer patients might sue because of overtreatment. A further report, in 2009, indicated that 20% of breast patients were overdiagnosed with ductal carcinoma in situ, a dormant non-invasive cancer that may be going nowhere. The pros and cons of screening programmes are now being widely debated.

Life expectancy is altogether different. Life expectancy in the USA is well down the league table. But if one removes fatalities from suicide, homicide and accidental injury, America has the longest life expectancy. This may be true, but it is rather like arguing that if Africa excluded malnutrition, AIDS and malaria, Africans would have a longer life expectancy. If you are dead, you are dead. These other causes of mortality have to be included, 'treated' if you wish. Suicide for instance is a disease of unease, mostly related to depressive illness. Homicide is endemic throughout America. It raises a larger philosophical question. Is the disparity of health between rich and poor a source of envy and frustration that contributes to an underlying malaise?

The debate between survival and cure has sometimes led to amusing exchanges. I recall one occasion at a surgical meeting in Boston where a physician argued that breast cancer is often incurable, some patients dying of the disease after decades. Dr Gilbert Fletcher from Texas, sitting in the front row, retorted, 'A 25-year survival may not be a cure, but it's a very good result for the patient.'

Innovation

One area where financial investment in America has yielded huge dividends is medical innovation. The USA is unarguably world leader in medical research and biotechnology, developing a wide range of pharmacological compounds and creating new medical products and devices.

Europeans, especially the British, would be quick to point out that the USA does not have a complete monopoly of discovery – witness penicillin. The story of the computed tomography (CT) scanner also aptly illustrates the situation. The CT scanner was discovered/invented by Godfrey Hounsfield working with EMI in England. It was the greatest development in imaging since Roentgen's discovery of X-rays. But the CT scanner was brought to the marketplace by American commercial 'know-how'. The same might be said for magnetic resonance imaging (MRI), jointly discovered by Paul Lauterbur in Illinois, USA, and Peter Mansfield in Nottingham, England, but made a reality in America.

Clinton's health plan

Reforming the fragmented health care system in the USA has been piecemeal over the years. In 1993, President Bill Clinton proposed a radical overhaul, with a comprehensive plan of universal health care for everyone. A key part of the plan involved forcing employers to provide health insurance for all employees, through competitive and closely regulated health maintenance organizations (HMOs). His wife, First Lady Hillary Clinton, was appointed to chair the Task Force entrusted with the plan. Hillary was not an elected official and became an easy target for the opposition. Republicans, other conservatives and the insurance companies opposed her plan vehemently. She failed to overhaul the system. It was subsequently derided and labelled 'Hillary Care'.

The Obama factor

In 2008, after eight years of George W Bush and the Republican Party, Barak Obama was elected. He made health care overhaul a prime objective of his presidency. 'What's the alternative?', he said.

Many in both parties agreed on the main points, such as having all Americans covered, and prohibiting insurance practices that refuse coverage to people with health problems. But there were disagreements on how to pay for it.

Obama's proposal to create a government-sponsored health programme to compete with private insurance companies proved an obstacle to bipartisan consensus on health reform. He has said, 'Doing nothing will cost us far more. Our deficits will be higher. Our premiums will go up. Our wages will be lower, our jobs fewer, our businesses will suffer.' Many demonstrated against his plans with placards: 'NObama', and 'No to socialism'. Socialism and liberalism have long been trashed of their meaning in America. They have become dirty words. Even Obama, defending his plans to an audience said, 'No one, certainly not me, is interested in a national health care system, like that in Great Britain. When you hear people saying socialized medicine, understand, I don't know anybody in Washington who is proposing that.'

Obama's proposals came at the time of a credit crunch when money was scarce. He suggested that some of the savings come from cutting back on excessive Medicare and Medicaid payments, and trimming federal payments to hospitals. He also proposed raising taxes on high earners, and limiting the value of deductibles they can claim, including charitable donations.

There was considerable support for his plan, but there was also widespread opposition. The pharmaceutical industry was cautious, especially regarding the proposal to switch to generic drugs rather than brand names. More worrying was the total silence on both sides about direct-to-consumer advertising of drugs on television. The Access to Medical Imaging Coalition was hostile, noting that the Obama plan 'would impair access to diagnostic imaging services, and result in patients delaying or foregoing life and cost saving imaging procedures'. Republicans accused Britain of trying to sell the NHS. But it was the other way around. Some Americans were 'bad mouthing' the NHS in the heated debate.

In an address to the American Medical Association (AMA), Obama told doctors that many unnecessary tests and procedures were conducted to hedge against malpractice suits. This has led to defensive medicine. He was careful, however, to stop short of capping malpractice awards, a decision that was met with derision by the doctors at the AMA.

Obama added, 'A big part of what had General Motors and Chrysler in trouble, were the huge costs they racked up providing health care insurance for their workers, costs that made them less profitable, and less competitive with automakers around the world. If we do not fix our health care system, America will go the way of GM, paying more, getting less, and going broke. It is a ticking time bomb.'

His plan had support in many quarters, especially from those who felt the private insurance companies were charging excessive premiums to patients. It was claimed that when competition was introduced, patients would have a choice between a government plan and a private plan, and would choose the government plan. But, as we have seen, the public option was doomed.

Health philosophy

Meanwhile little has been said, on either side of the Atlantic, about the cost savings that might be achieved by a change in the public attitude to health and disease. This calls for a philosophical shift that is not in vogue. Nonetheless, it is a truism that the conspicuous consumption of pharmaceutical pills and vitamins could usefully be replaced by a sensible diet and a little exercise. It is also true that too many patients, at the slightest sign of illness, are demanding unnecessary and expensive tests, backed by nervous physicians afraid of litigation.

Doctor substitutes

Analysing trends in health care in the USA reveals findings seen elsewhere. For instance, the division between doctors and paramedical personnel is gradually being eroded, for both pragmatic and financial reasons. Nurse anaesthetists complement medical anaesthesiologists. Prenatal, family planning and 'dysplasia' clinics, and some sexually transmitted disease clinics, which are government-funded, are mostly staffed by nurse practitioners. Physician assistants are filling in for doctors in remote rural areas. Again it has been noted that one reason health costs have risen sharply is the regulation requirement that prevents technicians without medical degrees from performing diagnostic and treatment procedures that carry little risk.

The futile pursuit

Most US health dollars are spent at the end of life. Estimates vary from 70% to 80%. The only firm figure comes from Medicare: 40% of payments are spent on the last 30 days of life. In their pursuit to extend life as long as possible, the wealthy have left the poor behind. Yet as already noted, there is an end point. The attempt to postpone indefinitely the wear and tear of ageing is a costly and futile exercise. An analogy that comes to mind is the dense spread of the Canadian population along the 49th parallel, in a forlorn attempt to get as far south as possible.

Driving up the costs of care

In a report on National Public Radio (NPR), entitled 'The Telltale Wombs of Lewiston, Maine', Alix Spiegel[1] tells the story of the extraordinary differences in the distribution of medical care in one region of New England. Jack Wennberg, a physician turned epidemiologist, was intrigued that so many women in the working class city of Lewiston, Maine, were having hysterectomies. If the rate continued, 70% of women in the community would have had a hysterectomy by age 70 years. Many reasons were advanced for the high rate, but none was satisfactory. Wennberg's team then amassed data over time on other health care differences in nearby Vermont. They found that people in one town would have five times more haemorrhoidectomies than in another town, only 30 miles away. The same was found for mastectomies, prostatectomies and back surgery. Children in one school system had a 75% chance of a tonsillectomy, whereas in another school the incidence was only 20%. In some areas, there was an epidemic of diagnoses.

In looking for an explanation, it was concluded that the differences were coming from the provider side. It was the doctors themselves who were using different thought processes. Again various reasons were advanced: older patients, heavy industry, lawsuits, medical training, and so on. Gradually – it took 20 years – it was conceded that money might also play a part. The US payment system rewards doctors for procedures. And the more complicated the procedure, the greater the payment. Needless to say, the doctors were not happy with the conclusion. Bob Keller, a spinal doctor in New England, quotes instrumented spinal fusion as a case in point. The procedure involves inserting metal rods to stabilize the spine. He says the operation literally took off, enabling surgeons 'to bill for putting in the screws, putting in the plates' and so on. He claims the procedure is probably no better than a less complicated and safer operation. Indeed, it can lead to the disabling 'failed back surgery syndrome'.

I spent some of my earlier years establishing radiotherapy in Maine, including part-time sessions in Lewiston. The practice in Lewiston was no different to elsewhere in the nation, whereby payments were made per radiation treatment, rather than per course of treatment. Fractionating treatment in small doses over an extended period of time resulted in higher fees. I don't believe that the system was abused, but the incentive was there. I do recall later a patient referred from Bermuda to a hospital on the outskirts of Boston. He had a basal cell cancer of the skin. Treatment was extended over six weeks, when it could have been delivered in one week, or exceptionally in one sharp treatment!

The fee-for-service principle encourages more tests, more surgery, more everything. Spiegel notes that most Americans assume more care is better. But this isn't necessarily so. Dr Elliott Fisher of the Dartmouth group estimates that almost one-third of the care given in the USA is not really helping people, and is driving up the costs of health care. Some have coined the phrase 'Less health care equals healthier patients'.

The Dartmouth Atlas of Health Care also found huge variations in the costs of end-of-life treatment. For instance, during the last six months of life, Medicare spent an average of $52,911 for UCLA patients and $28,763 for Mayo Clinic patients. Commenting on the study, Peter R Orszag, Director of the Congressional Budget Office, said, 'How can the best medical care in the world cost twice as much as the best medical care in the world?'

Dr Robert R Press, the Chief Medical Officer at New York University Medical Center, said that the Center was taking steps to tackle the problem. But he added, 'It's not an easy fix. We are dealing with a culture of physicians who have been very aggressive in their care, and a patient population that desire this type of treatment.'

Naomi Freundlich, the patient activist, suggests that 'entrenched interests – in screening, surgery, chemotherapy and other treatments associated with diagnosing more and more cancers – are impeding scientific evidence'. Barbara Ehrenreich, writing as a cancer patient, adds that she is suspicious of the oncologists, who saw their incomes soar in the late 1980s when they began administering and selling chemotherapy drugs in their 'ghastly, pink-themed *chemotherapy suites*'. She concludes that mammograms recruit women into chemotherapy, and the pink-ribbon cult recruits women into mammography.

The private practice segment of health care in the UK and elsewhere is also based on the fee-for-service principle. Intuitively, it is felt that similar conclusions might be drawn. This remains to be investigated.

The historic overhaul

The 23 March 2010 was a day that will live in American history books.[2,3] On that day, President Barack Obama signed the sweeping health reform legislation bill in the East Room of the White House. Yet the ideological and partisan battle raged on. The Senate Minority Leader, Mitch McConnell, said the Republicans have a plan of their own: 'Repeal and replace'.

The bill had been considered dead only two months previously, and was finally passed by a narrow vote of 219 to 212, with Republicans unanimous in opposition. It was predicted that the new provisions would cost $940 billion to implement over a decade. The legislation extended coverage to 32 million Americans who lacked it, and banned insurance companies from denying coverage on the basis of pre-existing medical conditions.

Representative John Clyburn of South Carolina, the top-ranking black member of the House said, 'This is the civil rights act of the 21st century'. The final obstacle to passage was cleared just a few hours before the vote when Obama issued an executive order that no Federal funds would be used for elective abortions. The measure satisfied Representative Bart Stupak of Michigan, who had lobbied for the amendment.

The reforms will be introduced gradually. In 2010, the uninsured will receive immediate access to coverage, and insurers barred from removing coverage when a person becomes ill. In 2011, insurers will be required to spend at least 80% of premiums on medical services. Over the following years, the taxpayer will have to foot the bill.

Too far, or not far enough

Amid the euphoria, there were voices that considered that the proposals only tinkered with the problem, and that the plans did not go far enough. In discussing Obama's speech beforehand, Arnold S Relman, Emeritus Professor of Social Medicine at Harvard, gave the President high marks for clearly stating the three fundamental goals of health care reform:[4]

1. Stabilizing and improving the health insurance of those already covered.
2. Providing affordable coverage for those not insured.
3. Achieving these objectives without increasing the deficit.

But Relman noted that the main drives of medical inflation are the fee-for-service payments to physicians. The incentives in the private medical market are to stimulate the delivery of more services. The business-oriented system drives up costs of health care, because the normal constraints between suppliers and consumers do not exist in medicine. He said, 'We will not control costs, without major changes in the way medical care is organized, delivered and paid for'. He deplored Obama's decision to abandon a strong public insurance option, 'in order to get something done now'. Relman added that the plan might work in the short term, but not for long.[5] He concluded that the inflationary forces will win, unless something is done to eliminate the profit motive from medicine, including licensing doctors so that they get a fixed salary each year, rather than, as now, making profits from prescribing more tests, procedures and visits, to increase their incomes. Sounds familiar.

References

1. Spiegel A. The telltale wombs of Lewiston, Maine. *National Public Radio (NPR)*, 8 October 2009.
2. Congress approves health care overhaul. *Associated Press*, 22 March 2010.
3. Tumulty K, Pickert K, Park A. Health care reform comes to America. The doctor will see you now. *Time*, 5 April 2010.
4. Relman AS. The folly of the middle course. Room for Debate Blog. *The New York Times*, 10 September 2009.
5. Relman AS. Waiting for the health reform we really need. *Tikkun*, 24 September 2009.

CHAPTER 6

The pursuit of health

Health education, promotion and protection

Ideally, prevention should eradicate the need for medical care. But prevention has been something of a Cinderella in medicine. Not because its importance isn't recognized, but because the urgency of acute illness demands immediate attention, whereas tomorrow's patients can wait until tomorrow. The ethos is changing, however. There is increased emphasis on early detection (now termed secondary prevention), and renewed interest in a healthy lifestyle. And life expectancy continues to increase in the Western World.

Chapter summary
- Health education, promotion and protection
- Screening and early detection
- The perils of idealism: doctor bashing, victim blaming
- Accidental death and injury
- The maverick view

I was the longest-serving member on the former Health Education Council (HEC) in Britain, lasting four terms of office, probably because I said it was better to prevent cancer than to try and treat it. That was true at the time, and remains so.

Cleaning up the water supply in the 19th century and alerting the present generation to the dangers of smoking remain classic examples of the dictum from the Temple of Delphi: 'Prevention is better than cure'. Today the HEC has been replaced by the Health Protection Agency, a more appropriate title.

Health education and protection had their origins in the past. Consider the apparently innocuous nursery rhyme:

> *Ring a ring of roses*
> *Pocket full of posies*
> *Atishoo, Atishoo*
> *All fall down.*

The verse allegedly referred to the plague. The ring of roses was the clinical sign, the posies the charm or talisman, the sneezing the respiratory symptoms, followed by collapse and death.

The English evangelist John Wesley recognized the value of simple hygiene when he coined the phrase 'Cleanliness is next to godliness'. This standard advice has been updated today as 'Now wash your hands'. Even as late as 1854, Chadwick, the pioneer of modern health legislation, had his Sanitation Bill defeated in Parliament. *The Times* of London thundered, 'We prefer to take our chance with cholera than be bullied into health.' No one now seriously questions the value of hygiene and sanitation in controlling cholera and typhoid fever. Fifty years ago in Ireland, health promotion played a vital role in the eradication of tuberculosis, emphasizing the value of mass radiography and fostering a more realistic attitude to the disease, bringing it out of the closet. But there are still battles to be won. Some in South Africa today still deny that AIDS is connected with HIV infection.

Efforts can also be misguided. Not that long ago, a prominent psychiatrist stated that 'bowel anxiety' was the commonest form of neurosis in Western society. It took health professionals many years to amend the message, and omit the earlier exhortations on inner cleanliness.

Again we need to ensure that the messages are consistent. At the time of writing, a study by an international cancer group found that people no longer accepted some messages because doctors often change their minds. By the end of the same week, a separate study stated that aspirin was no longer indicated as a preventive in cardiovascular disease, except in those with a previous history of heart trouble. For decades, thousands had been consuming low-dose aspirin every day!

Take tea drinking. The messages change every month. In June 2010, tea drinking increased the risk of rheumatoid arthritis. The previous month, nutritionists claimed tea was a healthier drink than water. Green tea prevents cancer. And so on. One man described his confusion: 'Doctors tell us not to worry when we are worried, and to worry when we are not worried.'

Yet health education remains important in conveying messages in many areas, from the value of immunization to the dangers of smoking. Critics claim that this approach is based on the biomedical model of disease, rather than the biosocial model of health. The problem is that models of the health disease spectrum are difficult to evaluate. For one thing, the parameters used to describe health are not precise mathematical functions, but abstract concepts that are difficult to define and often impossible to measure. Many of the causes of illness are unknown, and not related to previous health behaviour. Consequently, many diseases are not amenable to health education measures. Recognizing this limitation, we need to look at the entire range of normal health behaviour, and at ways and means of improving patterns of health. But there is an end point. Eventually the human protoplasm begins to burn out.

Meanwhile health educationalists and lifestyle gurus continue to lecture us on prevention along the traditional lines: Some of the following measures have been helpful in reducing premature mortality.

Diet

I used to tell medical students that the link between diet and cancer is a good news, bad news story. The bad news is that some of the things we eat are related to cancer. The good news is that we do not know what they are, so there is no use worrying about it. In many ways, that has not changed. We know in general terms what is good for you, and what is bad for you. But we are short on the specifics, and know little about the risks to individual patients. This is because the evidence comes from epidemiological studies of large numbers of people, and not from laboratory studies of chemical compounds. The causes of most diseases are multifactorial.

We know of course that obesity is bad, especially abdominal obesity associated with waist circumference. It is linked to diabetes, cancer and heart disease. And there is now some evidence that obesity is in our genes. We also know about the environmental factors. There is sugar in everything from cornflakes to ketchup.

The cholesterol saga has been going on for decades. It is recognized that there is 'good' cholesterol (high-density lipoproteins, HDL), and 'bad' cholesterol (low-density lipoproteins, LDL). We learn that consuming saturated fats is bad. It raises your LDL. Unsaturated fats, however, are good. They raise your HDL. The trick is to get the ratio right. But again it's not so much your diet, as your genes. So there has been a reappraisal: 'Welcome back to butter. And go to work on an egg.'

Then research uncovered a further complication: *trans fat*. This is a form of unsaturated fat, and you might expect it to be good. Not so. Although trans fats are unsaturated, they have been artificially hydrogenated, turning them into a more solid form. The National Academy of Sciences in the USA states that 'trans fatty acids are not essential and provide no known benefit to human health'. Indeed, they can be harmful. Nevertheless, the Academy has not recommended the elimination of trans fat from food, because it is useful for cooking. Moreover, it is naturally present in trace quantities in many animal foods. So the recommendation is that trans-fat consumption should be kept as low as possible. In Britain, NICE goes further and calls for trans fat to be eliminated from the food chain. It is also pressing for further reductions of salt and saturated fats, to help reduce the number of cardiovascular deaths.

The new solution, however, is statin drugs for everyone. Remarkably, as noted above, it took yet another study to show that the public don't know who to believe.

As for organic food, the Food Standards Agency, a government watchdog in the UK, reported in July 2009 that a scientific study showed that organic food contains no more nutritional value than conventionally produced food. The investigation was carried out by a team from the London School of Hygiene and Tropical Medicine, using data collected over 50 years. Organic groups were incensed by the findings. They said that the government didn't want to have a policy of making organic food available for everyone. The additional annual cost of buying organic food for a family of four is £1200.

A different debate is taking place in the USA, where one in four now buy organic. Although conventional food, such as apples, may have been treated with pesticide, there is no evidence that this causes cancer or other illness. On the other hand, big organic firms now use the same industrial-size farming and long-distance shipping methods as conventional farming. Food is often refrigerated and transported thousands of miles. Some claim that food grown in the neighbourhood is better. In the USA, local is the new organic. James McWilliams, a professor of environmental history in Texas, adds, 'We draw lines between organic and conventional food, but science doesn't draw those lines. They crisscross and we have people cherry-picking the data.' On balance, however, most agree that organic has the edge, especially in its treatment of animals.

The role of dietary supplements is also controversial. Vitamin C and D deficiency diseases, such as scurvy and rickets, are now extremely uncommon in the Western World, although vitamin B_{12} deficiency can still give rise to pernicious anaemia and subacute combined degeneration of the spinal cord. However, a meta-analysis of many studies in 2007 found that vitamin A and E supplements provide no health benefit, and may actually increase mortality (see Chapter 18). It is interesting too that the credit crunch of 2009 has meant a fall in the sales of vitamin pills. Many now opt for the cheaper choice of a simple nutritious diet.

Just when we thought that the benefits of vitamin supplements were exaggerated, along comes a study in September 2010, stating that high doses of B vitamins slow brain shrinkage and delay the onset of Alzheimer's disease.

A definitive study of the Mediterranean diet was published in the USA in 2009. The study of 23,000 people was led by Professor Dimitrios Trichopoulos, of the Harvard School of Public Health. It sounds as if the Professor's name is of Greek extraction, for not surprisingly his study confirmed the benefits of the classic Mediterranean diet. The study suggests, however, that not all the ingredients carry the same benefits. Eating larger amounts of fish and seafood, and low levels of dairy products, did little or nothing to lengthen lifespan. But eating large amounts of vegetables bathed in olive oil, plenty of fruit and nuts, and low amounts of red meat, increases your life span, especially if washed down with a glass or two of wine.

The report does not completely rubbish previous studies. Earlier studies did show that omega-3 oils (Greek again), the 'good' fatty acids from salmon and tuna, can slow the onset of dementia and lower the risk of prostate cancer.

Personally, I have always suspected that the warm Mediterranean climate plays a significant part in the healthy life. There is an old saying in physiology: 'Nude man is a tropical animal'. Nude woman too, for that matter. As for the regular diet of most people, the message has not changed – cut out the cakes, and curb the carbs.

Exercise

The value of exercise is a good example of the interplay between the factors involved. There is good scientific evidence that exercise reduces the incidence of cardiovascular disease and thereby lengthens life. Many years ago, one study showed that London bus conductors lived longer than bus drivers, presumably because they were more physically active. Similarly, another study showed that postmen delivering mail lived longer than postal sorters who sat at a desk all day. The same was true for sedentary and active civil servants. Exercise conditions the heart, but it has many other positive effects that are often overlooked. It increases muscle strength and stamina. It burns up calories and reduces weight and blood pressure. It goes further and curbs appetite, and even reduces dependence on alcohol and tobacco.

There is also evidence that physical inactivity and obesity are related to a higher incidence of colon cancer. The World Cancer Research Fund has noted that The Netherlands, where everyone is out on their bikes cycling to work and play, has one of the lowest colon cancer rates. Professor Jan-Willem Coebergh, of Erasmus University says, 'We can safely predict that increasing physical activity across Europe, to the level already achieved in The Netherlands, would be of substantial benefit.'

The psychological effects of exercise are equally important. It makes one mentally alert and sharpens the intellect. It calms and sedates nervousness and is better than tranquillizers. Athletes are well aware of its ability to induce euphoria, which is now known to be related to the release of beta-endorphins. At the end of the day, physical fatigue can ensure a good night's sleep without the need for sleeping tablets. The list goes on. So why isn't everyone out on the streets?

Smoking

It is difficult to say anything new about smoking, but smokers find the habit pleasurable. The message here is that smoking is a negative pleasure. Nicotine addicts are in a physiological state of negative nicotine balance. They have a constant craving for tobacco. Having placed themselves in this distressing state, the only way to obtain relief is to smoke. This pulls them up out of the negative state to the normal level. And this relief is pleasurable, but only in the relative sense. It is like banging your head against the wall. It is good when you stop.

There is another point that is often overlooked. Nicotine causes the addiction and the tar causes the cancers. *But it is the third factor, carbon monoxide, that is related to heart disease, especially cases of sudden death.* Recent studies have shown a dramatic drop in cardiac deaths with the decrease in smoking.

'We always knew a public smoking ban would bring rapid health benefits, but we have been amazed by just how big and how rapid they have been', said John Britton, Director of the UK Centre for Tobacco Studies at Nottingham University. Jill Pell, Public Health Professor at Glasgow University, estimated the sudden drop in heart attacks to be between 14% and 21% in various groups.

Coffee

Caffeine is also addictive, but for most people it is relatively harmless. The claim that it boosts your energy has been challenged by researchers at Galway University. Their studies suggest that serious coffee drinkers are caffeine-dependent. Drinkers who feel it lifts them up in the morning are merely reversing withdrawal symptoms. The same is true for food. When you are hungry with a voracious appetite, you are hypoglycaemic. Eating reverses the withdrawal symptoms. On the positive side, there is some evidence that coffee may delay the onset of Alzheimer's disease.

Alcohol

Not everyone who drinks alcohol becomes an alcoholic. But it remains a huge problem, and one that is increasing, especially in young people. How much health education can contribute to controlling the problem is arguable. The relatively low price of alcoholic drinks in supermarkets has been associated with a rise in binge drinking and alcohol-related hospital admissions. Politicians remain reluctant to intervene. And some stores have been selling vodka at less than cost, as a 'loss leader' to attract customers.

Aside from the dependency problem, there is a lesser effect that is worth noting. This is the relationship between alcohol and dieting. Alcohol has a triple effect. First, it has a calorific effect, albeit the so-called empty calories. Second, it has an aperitif effect, triggering the appetite. Third, and most importantly, it destroys willpower. I call it the 'Ah to hell factor'. You come home after a splendid dinner party, and head for the cookies in the refrigerator. Then there is the other problem, addiction. Although one glass of wine may be beneficial, two is borderline, and three not enough.

Education

Health education begins in the classroom. For health is a child's most valuable physical possession, more than brains, more than money, more than a prize in any field. Hanging on to it is vital. We have a responsibility to children to impart some basic information about the body they inhabit. About developing a healthy lifestyle. They need to know a little about human biology. For it is difficult to talk about smoking and lung cancer, venereal disease and sterility, alcohol and cirrhosis, without the child knowing the location and function of the lungs, the ovaries and the liver.

Risk perception

Much of health promotion has to do with risk perception. This may have little to do with the actual risks themselves, for instance the irrational fear of flying. But perception can be more important than reality. Risk perception is a function of many variables. Three can be readily identified: first, the probability of the event; second, the magnitude of the consequences; and third, the time delay before the onset.

The media

The press has an important role. Perhaps the most dramatic and sensational example was the canned salmon scare in Birmingham in 1978. Several elderly people in an old people's home died of botulism due to contaminated Alaskan salmon. Botulinum toxin is one of the most powerful poisons known to man. Within 24 hours of the news being broadcast, there was not a can of salmon sold in the entire nation, and the supermarket shelves were cleared completely. The message was 100% effective immediately.

But the media can also get it wrong. About the same time as the Birmingham scare, a tourist in Spain died of Legionnaires' disease in a town called Benidorm. The very name sounds like a sleeping tablet. The press picked up the story and created a fuss that amounted to panic. It had all the elements they wanted: a mystery illness threatening healthy British families in a foreign place. But the media didn't, and rarely do, report that 1000 travellers return from abroad each year to Britain with malaria, ten of whom die of the fever. An even larger number of young people return from these holidays with a sexually transmitted disease. Moreover, vast numbers scorch themselves on package sunshine holidays, and a significant number later develop the highly malignant melanoma.

Persuasion

In the end, health education involves changing behaviour. Seven levels of persuasion have been identified. There may be more.

1. Provision: The information is available for those who seek it out – e.g. travel advice on malaria and summer ailments.
2. Offer: Service advertised – e.g. family planning.
3. Invitation: Please avail yourself – e.g. cervical screening.
4. Encouragement: Attempting to convince people of the benefit – e.g. dieting and exercise.
5. Coercion: We will make you feel guilty if you decline – e.g. smoking in the presence of non-smokers.
6. Pressure: We will reward you if you do, and exert sanctions if you refuse – e.g. life insurance.
7. Compulsion: We have passed a law – e.g. rabies control, smoking in the workplace.

Lost in translation

The French have a different attitude to alcohol. Although cirrhosis of the liver was common in France in the past, one rarely saw drunks on the streets. Recently this has changed and binge drinking has arrived on the boulevards of Paris. The French also have a different definition of alcohol. Some years ago, a European Cancer Council in Brussels was devising a Cancer Code for Europe. I was the UK delegate. The French lady on the panel refused to classify beer and wine as alcohol. It was only much later I realized that 'alcool' in French refers exclusively to distilled spirits or hard liquor. The word was lost in translation.

Results

There is still some way to go in improving the health of the general population. But in the meantime there has been progress. The incidence of infant mortality has diminished. Smallpox has been eradicated. Heart attacks and acute ischaemic attacks have been halved, and the incidence of lung cancer has fallen, especially in men.

Screening and early detection

Early detection has been called secondary prevention. Screening for breast cancer, hypertension, cholesterolaemia and diabetes has lowered mortality. But screening tests need to be interpreted with caution, because of epidemiological bias. Two are important in cancer detection. They are length bias and lead-time bias:

- *Length bias* refers to the frequency of screening tests. Slowly growing tumours are more likely to be diagnosed, whereas faster growing tumours may arise in between the screening intervals, and can spread rapidly before detection.
- *Lead-time bias* refers to the time of diagnosis. Even if two patients die at the same time, and one is detected earlier because of screening, that patient may *appear* to have survived longer. This is due to the earlier countdown.

Broadly speaking, therefore, there are often two kinds of cancer: tiny aggressive tumours that spread rapidly, and may evade early detection; and larger indolent tumours that aren't going anywhere.

Meanwhile the search is on for better screening tests, and detection should improve by identifying hereditary risk factors in some diseases. Steady progress is being made in several areas. For instance, although the prostate-specific antigen (PSA) test in prostate disease is not specific for cancer, a better marker may be the heat shock protein Hsp27. Evidence suggests that its presence implies an aggressive form of the disease. Also interesting is the finding that a single PSA test at 60 years can distinguish between those with low levels, who are likely to have no further trouble, and those who need to be followed at regular intervals. Again a putative virus has been identified in some cases of prostate cancer, raising hopes of a possible vaccine. But more work needs to be done to confirm both of these findings.

Interestingly, screening for cervical cancer with the Pap smear test may eventually become redundant with the onset of vaccination against the papillomavirus, although this procedure has raised ethical concerns in some groups.

There are also economic and social difficulties. It would be possible for instance, to screen for the silent carriers of cystic fibrosis. But at present this would involve testing mass populations for a relatively small return. Beyond these advances, it is predicted we will eventually hit a wall with early detection, leaving additional tasks for fundamental research.

The perils of idealism: doctor bashing, victim blaming

Prevention appeals to politicians for economic reasons. The Health Education Council, however, began to go overboard. There was growing criticism of the so-called medical model. And the beginning of doctor bashing and, worse, victim blaming. It was your fault if you fell ill. You didn't wash your hands, you smoked cigarettes, you were promiscuous, you drank too much, you ate too much. Alas, victim blaming has entered the wider culture. The writer Barbara Ehrenreich quotes a classic example. A patient, responding to Barbara's blog, said that when she was diagnosed with advanced malignant lymphoma, a friend asked, 'What have you done to cause this?' The patient was speechless, then recovered to say, 'It's probably because I have such unsupportive friends.'

What disturbed me most, however, was the World Health Organization (WHO) definition of health: 'a state of complete physical and mental wellbeing, not *merely* the absence of disease'. It was the word *merely* that bothered me. The absence of premature disease by itself is a splendid goal. The WHO definition stopped just short of Thomas Jefferson's clause in the American Declaration of Independence: *'The pursuit of happiness'*. Or Franklin Roosevelt's New Deal slogan: *'A chicken in every pot'*. The Health Education Council was setting unrealistic goals. It was striving for an ideal world. Not something the NHS could deliver, let alone the medical profession.

There is nothing wrong with the pursuit of happiness, God knows. But incorporating it into a health programme by medicalization is overstretching (see later). Moreover, there are those who would argue that an element of stress can be productive. It is distress that one must combat.

In any event, the political undertone on the Health Education Council was too much for Margaret Thatcher, who promptly dissolved the body. She realized that it was an edentulous Quango. I predicted its demise when it failed to recognize the arrival of AIDS in its budget. Interestingly, the then Deputy Prime Minister, Willie Whitelaw, saw AIDS coming, and called it crudely 'that bugger's disease'. I was the only survivor on the Council and subsequently asked to continue on the new National AIDS Trust. But that too had an inauspicious start. First, it was set up as a government charity, which is an oxymoron, a contradiction in terms. And second because it appointed as its chairman the notorious Robert Maxwell. That is another story.

So health education has had its critics: from those who believe it doesn't go far enough, to those who believe it is fundamentally ineffective because of systemic contradictions in our society. The most damaging criticism, however, is that it is a middle class activity. Perhaps this is inevitable, since it is another way of saying that more intelligent people are more receptive to health messages. There is nothing intrinsically wrong in that. What we have to do is devise other means of getting through to other socio-economic groups. But we must not fall into the trap of assuming that alcohol and tobacco make life more tolerable for the underprivileged. In the end, they can make life more miserable. Or do they? Recall Will Fyffe's Scottish ballad, popularized by Gracie Fields, Danny Kaye and Eartha Kitt:

I belong to Glasgow,
Dear old Glasgow town;
But what's the matter wi' Glasgow,
For it's goin' roun' and roun'!
I'm only a common old working chap
As any one here can see,
But when I have a couple o' drinks on a Saturday,
Glasgow belongs to me!

Fyffe wrote the famous song after he encountered a genial drunk at Glasgow Central Station. The man was chatting about Karl Marx and John Barleycorn. Fyffe asked him, 'Do you belong to Glasgow?.' The man replied with a smile, 'At the moment, Glasgow belongs to me.' Not everyone approved of the lyric. Much to Fyffe's dismay, the famous Scottish troubadour Sir Harry Lauder refused to sing it.

Happiness

'Life is not a destination. It is a way of travelling.'

The pursuit of happiness is a noble goal. But it is not an end in itself – it is a by-product. Medicine can contribute to happiness, insofar as it enables people to enjoy good health. It is not the task of doctors, however, to prescribe happiness pills (see below). And alcohol and drugs are no solution. It is worth noting that in Scotland, the regional government has banned 'happy hours' in pubs.

Volumes have been written about happiness, sadness and depression. The subject is beyond the scope of this book. Nevertheless, hospitals could be more friendly places. Andy Burnham, the UK's Health Secretary under Labour in 2009, stated that the next phase of NHS reform will focus on improving patients' experiences, shifting the emphasis from medical care to the 'extras'. These softer aspects include cleanliness, attractive wards, friendly receptionists, the warmth of nurses, and doctors' bedside manners (again see later). Patients' satisfaction will be measured and hospital finances rewarded or penalized accordingly. The plan is admirable, so long as medical care is not downgraded in the process.

Accidental death and injury

There is one important area where health protection has a part to play, albeit mainly a legislative role. A primary task of medicine has been to prevent premature illness and death. The commonest cause of premature death is accidental. More than 3500 people are killed in one-quarter of a million road accidents in the UK every year. This is especially true of the younger generation. Road traffic accidents are so common, they are known in hospitals by the initials RTA. They account for about three-quarters of all accidental deaths between the ages of 15 and 24 years. Although young drivers make up only 7% of licence holders, they are involved in twice that percentage of accidents. Older drivers, incidentally, have recently been noted to have a disproportionate number of speeding tickets.

Deaths are only part of the horrific story. For every death, between two and three people are permanently disabled. Beyond that, the morbidity toll is enormous. In one UK county alone, Surrey, 6117 people were injured in 2007.

In the USA, deaths due to automobile accidents recently topped 43,000 in one year, far exceeding deaths due to falls, fire, accidental poisoning and drowning.

The numbers of RTAs have fallen over the years, owing to the use of seat belts and a number of innovations.

One more recent measure is a pioneering new road design developed in Sweden, and recently introduced in one section in Ireland. The so-called two plus one road is three lanes wide, with two lanes in one direction and one lane in the opposite direction. The direction of the two-lane section changes every mile or so, giving motorists repeated opportunities to overtake slow-moving vehicles. The innovation has a crucial extra safety feature, missing in most three-lane highways, namely a central crash barrier that separates oncoming traffic.

Yet there is still a considerable way to go in improving road safety. The number of accidents could be greatly reduced, not by a medical advance, but by a stroke of the pen. No government, however, has been willing or able to enact the draconian measures required – except one. I lived and worked in Bermuda for some years. The speed limit there is 21 mph, and motor vehicle accidents are extremely rare. Sadly, the accidents that do occur on the island are mostly among kamikaze riders on mopeds.

The first recorded death from a road accident was Mary Ward in Ireland on 31 August 1869. Mary fell under the steel wheel of her cousin's experimental steam car and died instantly from a broken neck. The Red Flag Act had come into force four years earlier, but didn't apply to private property. It limited speed in the country to 4 mph, and 2 mph in towns. The Act put an end to steam cars but the ICE (internal combustion engine) was just around the corner.

A personal anecdote indicates the scale of the problem today. A new motorway between Belfast and Dublin has transformed the journey between the two cities. The new highway culminates in a state-of-the-art tunnel, taking the motorist directly from Dublin Airport into the city in a few minutes, a journey that previously could take up to half an hour. One might have anticipated that drivers would be delighted with the innovation, and drive at a leisurely pace with a degree of caution. Not so. I travel regularly between the two cities, usually at the speed limit of 120 kph, marginally above 70 mph. Yet I am overtaken by a majority of drivers, well over the generous speed limit, some approaching the 'ton'.

On one occasion, a motorist passed me in a whirlwind. Further down the road, I came across a serious accident, probably not the same person, who no doubt was miles away. There were three ambulances, several police cars, a fire engine and multiple emergency personnel, perhaps a total of 20 people. Three or four would have been better engaged in monitoring the speeding motorists in the first place.

On another occasion, a 4 × 4 vehicle passed me in the underground tunnel, zigzagging across the lanes, ignoring the reduced speed limit and the two-chevron rule, and sped out of sight. The prospect of an accident and a fire engulfing the tunnel is an unimaginable catastrophe. It is a waste of time penalizing these drivers with points. They have to be taken off the road. Forever.

There is no need to clutter up our jails. Motorists who consistently defy the law are collectively as dangerous to society as sociopaths. Sadly, many are our best friends. The solution is simple. They must spend the rest of their lives on public transport. This is a double bonus, for the roads and for public transport. OK, I am a reasonable man: for a first offence, a severe warning. But two strikes and you are out!

Speeding, alcohol, young drivers and fatigue are common causes of RTAs. The greatest risk times are between 2 am and 6 am, when the roads are relatively empty, and between 2 pm and 4 pm, when they are busy. There is a case perhaps for lowering the speed limits during these danger hours. In fact, the speed limits need to be lowered all round, especially on secondary roads (which are much more dangerous than motorways) and during inclement weather. Maybe this need not be to the Bermuda level. It depends on what you consider an 'acceptable level of deaths'.

A 55 mph speed limit was introduced in the USA during the fuel crisis in the 1970s. It remained in force for nearly 20 years. Calls for its reintroduction have been met with outrage by many motorists. Yet the evidence suggests that it saved up to 4000 lives per year. But the serious opposition to a return of a 55 mph limit was summed up by one driver: 'I choose to drive at 80 mph in my SUV and will continue to do so regardless of the posted speed limit.' Curiously, truck drivers are said to welcome a revival of the so-called 'double-dime' limit, because of the spiralling costs of diesel.

Purists will rightly argue that the word 'accident' is a misnomer. Accidents are no accident. An accident, by definition, is an unforeseen event without an apparent cause, something that occurs by chance. In most road accidents, the cause is obvious. They do not occur by chance.

The end of trauma on the roads would not spell the end of medicine. It would, however, reduce the large number of victims in emergency medicine and intensive care. It would also considerably reduce the subsequent workload in orthopaedics, vascular surgery, prosthetics and rehabilitation medicine, and the long-term toll on mental health and social welfare.

The UK government is currently considering proposals to reduce speed limits in urban and residential areas from 30 mph to 20 mph, especially near schools. A 15-year study by The London School of Hygiene and Tropical Medicine, published in the *BMJ* in December 2009, found that reducing the speed limit to 20 mph cut road deaths by over 40%, including children and cyclists. But speed limits are only as good as their enforcement. Speed cameras cannot detect obscured or dirty registration plates, and you cannot have a policeman on every corner.

An alternative measure is being tested on a bus by Transport for London. Intelligent speed adaption (ISA) uses a new digital speed limit map of the city. The technology prevents vehicles speeding. In the override mode, you cannot accelerate once you reach the speed limit. If tests are successful ISAs may be introduced for London taxis as well. This measure has added benefits in that it will lower emissions, reduce speeding points, penalty notices and fines.

Speed governors for cars have been available for many years, but never seriously considered by legislators. Tom Edwards, the BBC London Transport correspondent, has road-tested the ISA device. He says that it works 99% of the time. He adds that there are two modes to the gadget, and it can be disabled at the touch of a button (although many feel that this defeats its purpose). Edwards says, however, 'It is unlikely there will ever be the political will to make this device compulsory.'

The Parliamentary Advisory Group for Transport Safety (PACTS) has called the death toll on roads 'a scandal of tolerance'. Cathy Keeler, of BRAKE, a charity that supports the bereaved from road deaths, says the epidemic strikes indiscriminately, devastating communities. 'If the same numbers were killed on planes or trains, there would be a national outcry, and a rush to implement policies to stop the carnage.' There is a fatalism about it all. The Director of PACTS, Robert Gifford, says that we need to puncture some of the myths around cars: 'The automobile has two attractive features, autonomy and mobility. The trouble is everyone wants both.'

There is a looming battle ahead. Nothing will happen quickly. It took decades before smoking in public buildings was prohibited by law. Equally, it took many years before seat belt legislation was enacted. With road accidents, saving a few lives might arguably be worth the legislation. How about saving hundreds, nay thousands?

Meanwhile, one cannot be optimistic. No sooner was the new coalition government in office in Britain in May 2010 than Philip Hammond, the new Transport Secretary, in a populist move, promised to end the 'war on motorists'. He pledged to scrap public funding on speed cameras. Many were dismayed with his statement, including the Automobile Association (AA). The previous year, the London Transport Commissioner and the Metropolitan Police Commissioner both noted that funding speed cameras had prevented 400 people a year being killed or seriously injured in the capital. Hopefully, Hammond may have misread the populist mood, and the feelings of law-abiding motorists, who want to rid the roads of homicidal boy racers.

Looking far ahead, another approach may be developed. Nissan, the automobile manufacturer, has tested a robotic car that mimics the movement of shoals of fish. Fish use 'lateral line sense' when travelling side by side, to avoid collisions. No doubt, we will have to wait many decades before the technique is adopted on our highways. Until then, doctors will be involved in stitching together the wounded. One local woman I heard about as I write will not be salvaged. She was a young mother and was cut in two in a collision, one half of her torso found a hundred yards away from the other half. The driver of her car was also killed. Police inform me he was out of control and seriously over the speed limit.

The maverick view

> 'Many times man lives and dies
> Between his two eternities.'
> W B Yeats

The benefits of health education, protection, screening and early detection are well documented. At the same time, some argue there is a downside. The ritual of the annual check-up is no substitute for healthy living. Achieving a balance is difficult. On the one hand, getting the 'all clear' is no guarantee that all is clear. There may be problems below the level of detection, or problems one can do little about. Second, there is the prospect of creating an epidemic of hypochondrias. We are becoming preoccupied with ourselves. A new condition has been described in healthy patients undergoing tests. It has been called '*Waiting for the results syndrome*'.

We need to keep a sense of perspective. Although there is a place for health education, we must not adopt the frantic approach that is sweeping North America, and threatening our shores. Lewis Thomas, the former Director of the Sloan Kettering Cancer Institute in New York, and sometime essayist in the *New England Journal of Medicine*, caricatured the scene in the tradition of Mark Twain. His views can be paraphrased for Britain:

> '*Squash is more than a sport. It is a rigorous discipline, a form of collective physiotherapy. Jogging is done by groups of people, out on the streets every day, in underpants, moving in solid files, hoping by this to stay alive. Meditation may be good for the soul, but it is even better for the blood pressure. We must not become obsessed with health. We do not seem to be seeking exuberance in living, as much as staving off failure and dying. We have lost confidence in the human body.*
>
> '*The new consensus is that we are badly designed, intrinsically fallible, vulnerable to disease. This new view seems to have been initiated in the advice columns of our magazines and media, especially in the USA. Get a check up, go on a diet, make sure it is organic, meditate, have some surgery. Take two vitamin tablets with water, preferably spring water. If boredom persists see your doctor.*'

It is extraordinary that we have become convinced of our bad health when the facts suggest the opposite. Out of a population of over 60 million in Britain, only 1% died last year, which isn't bad, not at all a discouraging record, once you accept the fact of mortality itself. So we are, in real life, in the Western World, a reasonably healthy people. Thomas adds 'Far from being ineptly put together, we are tough durable organisms, ready for most contingencies. The new danger is that if we become obsessed with the health ethic, we may become neurotic, living gingerly and worrying unnecessarily.'

So it is important to make the plea that although health education is a serious pursuit, we must never take ourselves too seriously. If, on the one hand, complacency is our enemy, on the other, a lack of humour, an inability to laugh at ourselves, at our central dilemma, could be our downfall. Not least in the eyes of those we are most trying to convert.

References

1. Lowry S. Public cancer education. *Health Education Journal* 1979; **38**: 23–9.
2. *Dietary Reference Intakes for Energy*. National Academy of Sciences Report, 2002.
3. Silberner J. Statins may help already low cholesterol levels. *National Public Radio (NPR)*, 11 November 2008.
4. Elliott V. Organic food has no extra health benefits. *The Times*, 30 July 2009.
5. Kluger J. What's so great about organic food? *Time*, 18 August 2010.
6. Cloud J. Eating better than organic. *Time*, 2 March 2007.
7. Devlin K. Wine, fruit and olive oil, a recipe for long life. *The Daily Telegraph*, 24 June 2009.
8. Leake J. Heart attacks plummet after smoking ban. *The Sunday Times*, 13 September 2009.
9. Lowry B. Pioneering road aims to slash death count. *The News Letter (Belfast)*, 7 November 2007.
10. Plans to cut traffic speed limits. *BBC News*, 21 April 2009.
11. Speed limit device tested on bus. *BBC News*, 11 May 2009.
12. Massey R. Labour's 13-year war on the motorist is over. Tories pledge to halt the rise of speed cameras, road pricing, and cowboy clampers. *Daily Mail*, 14 May 2010.
13. Thomas L. The Health Care System. *New England Journal of Medicine*, 11 December 1975; **293**: 1245–6.

CHAPTER 7

Malpractice and defensive medicine

Medical scandals

Chapter summary
- Medical scandals
- Clinical acumen and medical evidence
- Disagreeable doctors
- Litigation and defensive medicine

Critics have had no difficulty finding an excuse for doctor bashing. There have been many medical scandals. Indeed, the catalogue of crimes and misdemeanours has been so many and manifest that one is tempted to ask how did medicine get away with it for so long? Today, the apparent increase in scandals may be mostly due to increased scrutiny, accountability and publicity.

One of the earliest scoundrels was Dr Harvey Crippen, who poisoned his wife with hyoscine and went off to Canada with his lover, only to be apprehended on the ship by wireless telegraph. (There is now some intriguing DNA evidence that the corpse in Crippen's cellar was not his wife, but a man!)

Then there was Dr John Bodkin Adams, a Northern Ireland medical graduate, much to the dismay of the Queen's University Dean, John Henry Biggart. Adams practised family medicine in Eastbourne, England. One hundred and sixty of his patients died suspiciously. Many were elderly dowagers and 132 patients left him money or items in their will. He was tried and acquitted for the murder of one patient, but was found guilty of prescription fraud, lying on cremation forms and failing to keep a dangerous drug register. He was removed from the medical register in 1957 but reinstated four years later.[1]

There was also the case of James Wishart in Bristol. He didn't poison anyone. But too many of his young cardiac patients died after surgery and he was hounded. Many believe he was the victim of a witch-hunt and made a scapegoat.

Professor Roy Meadow and Dr David Southall were not the first paediatricians to be severely criticized for giving exaggerated evidence in child abuse trials. There was the case of Dr Marietta Higgs in Cleethorpes years previously, who was harassed by the media for similar reasons. She allegedly remains unrepentant (see 'Clinical acumen and medical evidence' below). Conversely, in the subsequent infamous Baby P trial, where the child died following extreme abuse, the doctor who failed to diagnose the child's injuries, Dr Sabah Al-Zayyat, was under investigation.

Consider also the case of Dr Andrew Wakefield and the controversy surrounding MMR vaccine and autism. His *Lancet* paper says: '*We did not prove an association between MMR vaccine and the syndrome*'. Yet Wakefield went on to suggest there was a link, and that was sufficient to set off a scare about the vaccine. As there was no evidence of a link, 10 of his 12 *Lancet* coauthors withdrew their support, and the journal retracted the paper. Meanwhile, there has been a drop in the number of vaccinations in Britain and the USA. Wakefield was given time on the *Oprah Winfrey Show*, and was involved in a clinic supported by celebrities in Texas. He was subsequently discredited by the General Medical Council, and struck off in May 2010, but the damage had already been done.[2]

Harold Shipman was in a different category, the most notorious physician of all. A serial killer, Shipman was found guilty of 15 murders, although over 200 killings were ascribed to him. Following his conviction, the legal structure of health care and medicine in Britain was reviewed.

There were lesser rogues: Dr Allan Zarkin, a New York obstetrician, who was so pleased with his surgical skills that in 1999 he carved his initials on a patient's abdomen. Nearer home, there was Dr Michael Neary, a gynaecologist in Ireland, who allegedly performed an excessive number of hysterectomies without consent:[3] some say it was a radical form of birth control.

There is also the problem of exploitation. Recently, a friend informed me of a fellow passenger on a cruise liner, who attended the ship's doctor with a trivial complaint, looking for an aspirin. The doctor ordered a battery of tests costing several thousand pounds. The patient only had a sore throat.

I believe that most doctors are competent and many excel. But there are still those who fall short, and a few who the late Professor Harold Rogers described as a 'stain on the profession'. This is true in every walk of life, in commerce, in law, certainly in politics, and even in the church. Weeding out the bad apples is difficult. However vigilant, there will always be some who slip through the net. And the bad cases attract a triad: notoriety, publicity and litigation.

Clinical acumen and medical evidence

The cases of the paediatricians mentioned above demonstrate that doctors often make diagnoses using clinical acumen. This is on the basis of diagnostic probability. They are correct say 70–80% of the time. But criminal law demands as close to certainty as possible, beyond all reasonable doubt, say 99%. And even when doctors are 99% right, they can still be wrong. Spontaneous regression of incurable disease is a rare but recognized phenomenon. I have only seen one case in my entire career. I suspect most of my colleagues have seen none. And of course the same is true in law. In rare cases, innocent men have gone to the gallows. Not surprisingly, paediatricians are now reluctant to diagnose childhood abuse, even where the evidence is clear, but short of certainty.

The case of Ernest Saunders[4] illustrates another problem for 'expert' medical witnesses. Saunders was one of the Guinness Four fraudsters convicted in 1991. He was sentenced to five and a half years in prison, later reduced to two and a half years. But he is better remembered for the diagnosis of his dementia, a condition that saw him released after serving only 10 months. His doctors said that Saunders' mental condition was so poor that he couldn't remember three numbers backwards, or the name of the American President. An eminent neurologist demonstrated, with the help of flip charts and brain scans, that Saunders' brain was abnormally small for a man of his age. It had shrunk to a level seen in Alzheimer's disease or dementia. One tabloid reporter in court whispered, 'Not even Ernest is capable of conning a brain scan.' Shortly after, Saunders was released on compassionate grounds.

Within months, Ernest made a miraculous recovery and was back in business, as a consultant to Carphone Warehouse, advising a publicity company, and leading a consortium to buy the football club Queen's Park Rangers.

The medical diagnosis of dementia in Mr Saunders was extraordinary. The case reveals the unreliability of medical evidence in some situations, and the damage it does to the credibility of the medical profession. On the other hand, the Saunders case enhanced the reputation of the defending barrister, the late Richard Ferguson QC.

Medical advice can also take on a political dimension, as was seen in the case of the Lockerbie bomber. Abdelbasset Ali Mohmed al-Megrahi was released from jail on compassionate grounds, with only three months to live. But he confounded the doctors' prognosis, and was still alive well over one year later. Oncologists recognize that predicting the outcome in cancer patients is tricky, especially in prostate malignancy. It can fool physicians. Only when the patient is moribund, no longer eating or drinking, semi-comatose and Cheyne–Stokes breathing, is it relatively safe to say that life is drawing to a close.

Disagreeable doctors

When Alexander Pope wrote the lines 'Who shall decide when doctors disagree', he had in mind conflicting opinions. He was not thinking of violent confrontation, and certainly not of the fisticuffs. That, however, is what happened in an operating theatre in Belgrade in 2007. Two Serbian surgeons, Spasoje Radulovic and Dragan Vukanic, were doing an appendectomy on a patient. As reported in the *Reader's Digest* (June 2007, p. 69), Dr Radulovic made disparaging remarks about Dr Vukanic's professionalism. Dr Vukanic proceeded to pull Dr Radulovic's ear, slapped him on the face and walked out of the room. Dr Radulovic abandoned the sleeping patient and quickly followed him. According to the anaesthetist, fisticuffs ensued, resulting in a fractured finger, split lip, bruises and loose teeth. The patient remained blissfully unaware of the violence, while another staff member stepped in and completed the surgery. Hopefully, this is an unusual occurrence, even in Serbia.

Litigation and defensive medicine

Litigation has led to defensive medicine and the downgrading of the profession. The former Lord Chief Justice of Northern Ireland, Robert Carswell, took a kind but chilly look at this in his address to the Ulster Medical Society,[5] 'Doctor knows best'.

Medical litigation is widespread in the USA. There are said to be more malpractice lawyers than doctors in some areas. In a few states, there are only a few doctors practising obstetrics and gynaecology. In one reported instance, a doctor has a notice on his office door stating he has no financial means. No point in suing him, all his assets are in his wife's name.

Because policing the profession was relatively lax in the past, the pendulum has now swung the other way in Britain. The medical authorities are now over-zealous, eager not to be accused of a whitewash. A patient can accuse a doctor under a cloak of anonymity, and the doctor is tried in the court of public opinion. An acquittal may come too late. The professional damage has already been done.

There is growing concern that some patients may be pursuing trivial cases, and that many doctors are being put under unendurable stress. In the year 2003–4, nine of 215 doctors undergoing 'fitness to practise' died. The Wikipedia[6] site on the General Medical Council carries the comment, 'The suicide rate among doctors undergoing GMC Fitness to Practise is very high, fuelling doubts about their sentences being proportionate and fair.'

It is claimed that in five years' time there will not be a single doctor in Florida without a case pending against him – which recalls a comment the late Professor Macafee made to our student group. He said that a gynaecologist who has not accidentally cut a ureter hasn't done much gynaecology. Perhaps a physician in Florida who has not been sued isn't much of a physician. All this of course drives up the malpractice premiums, which in turn are passed back to the patients. The size of some of the financial awards has been a further incentive to sue the doctor. As noted already, even Obama has declined to cap these awards.

The most common cause of litigation in the USA is failure to diagnose, specifically failure to detect breast cancer. As already noted, fear of being sued has led to over-diagnosis, not only of breast cancer but also prostate cancer and malignant melanoma. Indeed, some epidemiologists claim that the incidence of breast cancer has gone up by 40%, but the mortality has hardly changed – evidence that many so-called malignancies are clinically benign.

As a result, litigation is now leaning the other way, and there is a move to sue doctors for over-diagnosis and over-treatment. *Under-diagnosis or over-diagnosis, either way it is a lose–lose situation.*

In fairness, it is not only the fear of litigation that may influence the doctor to over-treat someone. No physician deliberately wants to leave a patient at risk by withholding treatment. Thus, many elderly people with indolent tumours that aren't going anywhere are being subjected to therapy with unpleasant side effects that diminish the quality of life. Many physicians agree that, in these cases, the doctor is 'treating himself'.

pump inhibitor omeprazole. Many of these drugs can be obtained over the counter, without consulting a doctor.

The trend towards less surgery has also been seen in benign prostate hyperplasia. Open prostatectomy, a bloody operation, has almost disappeared, replaced by the simpler transurethral resection (TUR) of the prostate. And even this procedure is often postponed until medication with finasteride has been tried for patients presenting with retention of urine.

Tonsillectomy, once termed 'the tonsillar pillars of gold', has been in decline for years, although new surgical procedures, such as cochlear implants for deafness, have emerged. Meanwhile, the cause of tinnitus, a debilitating ringing in the ears afflicting millions of people, has been elucidated. Damage to hair cells in the inner ear prompts auditory areas of the brain to fill in the missing sound, creating phantom noise.[1] The hope is that a drug may be devised to block the feedback signals producing the noise.

One procedure where the demand for surgery has remained fairly constant is the repair of inguinal hernia. Interestingly, within the NHS, it has been suggested that patients should live with the inconvenience until it becomes symptomatic. Only then should herniorrhaphy be considered. Jonathan Meakins, former Nuffield Professor of Surgery at Oxford, has recommended watchful waiting in early cases.[2] If the patient is symptom-free, he believes there is no point in running the 20% risk of post-herniorrhaphy pain syndrome (PHPS).

Although surgery has been in retreat in some areas, it has rebounded in others, with the emergence of 'spare-parts surgery'. Leading the field is hip replacement, followed by developments in cardiovascular surgery, ophthalmology, and especially transplant surgery.

At the sharp end of surgery is what *Time* magazine calls the invincible cancers: lung, pancreas, bladder and brain. Two things have happened in lung cancer. The decrease in smoking has led to a fall in the incidence of the disease in men. Second, a gene has been identified whereby those who smoke and have the defect are very likely to develop the disease. A similar genetic defect has been found in bladder cancer. Those who smoke and have the gene allegedly have 100% chance of developing bladder cancer.

Pancreatic cancer, however, remains stubbornly resistant to any form of treatment. Whipple's by-pass palliative operation is often the only thing surgery has to offer. The gliomas of the brain are equally resistant to treatment. Neither of these diseases appears to have a surgical future.

Nanosurgery

Philip Sharp, a Nobel Prize-winning cancer researcher at the Massachusetts Institute of Technology (MIT), has devised a different strategy for his new $100 million cancer research centre in Boston. He has put together a multidisciplinary team of biologists, chemists and engineers, skilled in nanofabrication. Professor Sharp is optimistic and enthusiastic: '*It's MIT,*' he says, '*We shake and bake!*' One of the first developments in Boston is a device using a nanoparticle to deliver chemotherapy in prostate cancer. The nano-weapon has three constituents: first it contains the warhead or killing agent, a common chemotherapeutic drug, docetaxel; second, it is enclosed in a 'stealth coating' to avoid rejection by the body's immune system; third, it has a homing device, targeting ligands, that directs the warhead to the cancer cells. Testing is already underway.

Meanwhile, an important development in surgery in recent years has been minimally invasive keyhole surgery, the laparoscopic approach. One advantage of this is faster recovery and shorter hospital stays. Alongside this are the peripheral surgical skills, endoscopy, angioplasty, and the insertion of stents and prostheses. Around the corner is the promise of robotics.

Robotics

Unlike keyhole surgery, in which the anatomical organs are displayed in two dimensions on a flat screen, robotic surgery is viewed through stereoscopic lenses, giving a three-dimensional image (see Colour Plate 2). In prostatectomy, for instance, the delicate structures on the pelvic floor are easily distinguished. Moreover, the machine eliminates any tremor in the operator's hands. One problem with robotics, however, is the absence of haptic feedback, the sensation of touching and feeling the different types of tissue. But this is offset, to some extent, by a device known as 'force constraint', which blocks the operator from damaging normal structures. Also under investigation is 'augmented reality', a means of enhancing not only the anatomical detail, but also the function of the tissues.

Ahead are two other developments: surgery by mouth, and intraoperative simulation. It may soon be possible to avoid surgical excisions altogether, and allow a snake-like robot to enter through a body orifice. Beyond that is the final taboo – simulating the surgical procedure in advance, and programming the robot to complete the task by itself.

General surgery

The general surgeon began to disappear some time ago, as the specialty fragmented into a number of subspecialties, mostly based on organ systems. These include neurosurgery, thoracic surgery, urology, orthopaedic surgery, otorhinolaryngology, and so on. Even within these subspecialities, further subgroups have evolved – for instance orthopaedists specializing in the knee, as opposed to the hand, and ophthalmologists specializing in the anterior segment of the eye, and others the retina.

The 'dentalization' of surgery

A question to consider is whether each of these specialties requires the long and arduous training so far entailed? An orthopaedic surgeon would not consider attempting cataract surgery, and vice versa. At what point do their training programmes diverge? A later section in this book considers the evidence that mental powers peak at 22 years, and begin to decline at age 27! Can we fast-track the surgical training programme to utilize these men and women during their most productive years, along the lines of training in dental surgery – the 'dentalization' of surgery? The dental model has been tried and tested for over a century. Is the surgical technologist such a far-fetched idea?

The Barraquer Dynasty

The Spanish ophthalmologist Joaquin Barraquer has inadvertently shown what can be achieved with early training. Joaquin is the son of Ignacio Barraquer and grandson of Jose Antonia Barraquer, an ophthalmic dynasty spanning five generations.

Jose Antonia instructed his son Ignacio in the use of a microscope, about the same time Pasteur was studying microbes. Ignacio in turn introduced his own son, Joaquin, to ophthalmology. From the age of 11, the boy spent many hours in the laboratory and with patients. *By the time he was 13, he was scrubbed up and assisting his father at cataract surgery.* Joaquin went on to become one of the most distinguished ophthalmologists of his generation, venerated in The American Society of Cataract Surgeons Hall of Fame.[3]

Cataract surgery is one of the most intricate surgical procedures and also one of the most successful. The Barraquers have shown what can be done with early exposure to surgical skills. An ophthalmic colleague assures me that he could train his own son to be a competent eye surgeon by the age of 20. Why then are we waiting?

The changing scene

The 'dentalization' of surgery may be a controversial concept, even preposterous in some circles, but who can predict what may transpire in the decades ahead? At present, there are 57 medical subspecialties – and still expanding. The fragmentation of medicine and surgery is inevitable. The wind of change may not be so far away. Already Texas Tech University in the USA is planning a three-year MD degree programme[4] for students who want to enter family medicine in an accelerated course (see later). Whether this could be extended to include some surgical subspecialties remains to be seen. One specialty has already emerged. The podiatric surgeon is not medically qualified yet performs invasive surgery on the foot (Chapter 18).

Before then, scientific advances will make further inroads into medicine and surgery. At present 50,000 hip replacements are performed in Britain each year. Experimental work already suggests that hip prosthesis may be superseded by stem cell therapy. Scientists in Southampton have taken purified cells from bone marrow in the patient's pelvis. The immature stem cells were then mixed with 'cleaned' bone from another patient. Dead tissue was then removed from the acetabulum, and the cavity was filled with a mixture of stem cells and donated bone. So far, half a dozen patients have been treated, with only one failure. It is too soon to predict the future of this procedure, but it sounds promising.

A similar procedure has been performed on a 30-year-old woman in Spain, who had tuberculosis of the trachea, or windpipe. A donor windpipe was taken from a patient who had recently died. The cells were then washed away using strong chemicals, leaving only an inert tissue scaffold. This was then repopulated with the patient's own stem cells, cultured in Bristol, which eventually grew around the donor windpipe. The European team believe such tailor-made organs could become the norm. But the new technology does not preclude surgery. The surgeon is part of a new team.

In another advance, the breast cancer gene *BRCA1* has been identified and genetically excised in one family with the abnormality. Similar genetic flaws have been identified in ovarian cancer and colon cancer that may permit the selection of tumour-free offspring.

The interplay of environmental factors can also reduce the need for surgical and medical intervention. Smoking restrictions have led to a reduction in lung cancer and sudden cardiac deaths. Exercise and weight reduction can lower the incidence of colon cancer. Prevention is still the golden goal of medicine.

Notwithstanding the advances that will be made, and the frontiers that will be crossed, there are some areas where surgery will endure. The acute abdomen remains the classic surgical emergency. It is difficult to envisage a robot handling this problem in the middle of the night. Moreover, trauma and haemorrhage, like the poor, will always be with us. 'Band Aid' surgery will survive indefinitely.

The bedside 'badside' manner

Many deplore the loss of the bedside manner and the absence of compassion in some physicians and surgeons. The problem is considered elsewhere in this treatise. There is one surgeon that I know of who specializes in a specific but rare problem of the spine. I cannot say who he is, or even which country he works in, but his ability and skills are unmatched. He is difficult to see because of his fame in the field. The only problem is that the man is unable to communicate. Apparently, it is worse – he is gruff, distant, almost autistic.

Patients are filtered through to him and the preoperative work-up done by others. If he agrees to tackle your problem, you are wheeled into the operating room, already unconscious, and he sets about resolving your problem. Is this the man you want to see, or literally not see? For he is probably going to cure you where everyone else has failed.

It is possible to be kind, considerate, talented and skilled. But you can't always have everything. The autistic surgical savant occasionally has his place.

References

1. Rauschecker JP. Imaging reveals how brain fails to tune out phantom sounds of tinnitus. *Science Daily*, 23 June 2010.
2. Lambert V. Why are men being refused surgery for their hernias? *Daily Mail*, 23 June 2009.
3. American Society of Cataract and Refractive Surgery: Hall of Fame Award, Joaquin Barraquer, 2003.
4. Jaschik S. Will medical schools join the 3-year degree trend? *USA Today*, 25 March 2010.

CHAPTER 10

The enigma of the brain

Understanding the workings of the mind has baffled doctors, scientists and others for generations. The extent of medicine's involvement is constantly changing. For instance neuro-psychiatry was once classified as a single specialty. Today, the distinction between the two fields is clear-cut. Diseases such as multiple sclerosis, syringomyelia and motor neurone disease belong in neurology. Thought disorders such as schizophrenia belong in psychiatry.

Chapter summary

- Autism
- Savants
- Synaesthesia
- Dyslexia
- Mental illness

Autism-spectrum disorders are less well understood. Views differ. Some mental health workers are seeking a cure. Others believe autism should be tolerated as a difference, and not treated as a disorder.

Dyslexia is less controversial. It is primarily a learning disorder concerned with reading difficulty and spelling. As such, it is an educational deficiency rather than a neurological disease.

Some other definitions are helpful. A prodigy is a brilliant child who has acquired adult skills at an early age, whether it be in music, mathematics or art. This precocious overdevelopment is often followed by an outstanding career in later life. The recognition of genius in whatever field is self-evident. It is not simply a matter of a stratospheric IQ. The defining characteristic of genius is creativity.

As with many branches of medicine, the normal merges with the abnormal, and the dividing line between mental health and mental illness is blurred. It is a continuum. Peering into the future of psychiatry and the role of the physician requires a closer look at some of these conditions.

Autism

Autism is a developmental brain condition characterized by impaired social interaction, communication and imagination. Those with the disability have said that the world is a mass of people, places and events, which they struggle to make sense of, and which can cause stress and anxiety. It may sometimes manifest itself by restricted and repetitive behaviour.

Caring for children with autism is a huge task for parents. One mother relates how her child had a convulsion, and subsequently stopped talking, eating and sleeping and lost all eye contact. These children regress into their own world and often become hypersensitive to noise.

Many measures have been tried, including biomedical intervention, detoxifying children through supplements and probiotics, diet, secretin, hormone, speech therapy, and behaviour therapy. One mother who runs a support group says, 'These children are being treated like cabbages. We can do better than that.'

There is also some evidence that children with autism spectrum disorder (ASD) have a pattern of gut microbes that can be detected in urine samples. The hope is that the chemical fingerprint will permit earlier diagnosis, and prompt treatment before permanent damage has been done.

Asperger syndrome is part of the autism spectrum. People with the condition find it harder to read the signals that most of us take for granted. They have some difficulty in communication, although fewer problems with speaking. It is often described as a hidden disability, in that they may have few outward signs of the condition. Those with Asperger syndrome are not incapacitated to the same extent as those with full-blown autism, although they may have problems with dyslexia and attention-deficit hyperactivity disorder (ADHD). With support and encouragement, they can often lead full and independent lives.

There is an interesting body of evidence that children with special needs, behavioural problems, autism-spectrum disorders, and even dyslexia, benefit from the therapeutic power of being around horses.[1] Veterinary scientists have known for many years that only three animals have been domesticated: the dog, the cat and the horse. Even our genetically related primates have not been domesticated on this scale. The dog and the cat have been intensively studied, but the horse hardly at all. Academics at Southampton University are expected to report shortly on a remarkable relationship between horses and emotionally disturbed children (see later).

The horse's genetic code[2]

There is now some genetic evidence to support the therapeutic empathy between horses and emotionally disturbed children. A complete blueprint of the domestic horse's genetic code has revealed remarkable similarities with that of *Homo sapiens*. Horses suffer from more than 90 hereditary diseases common to humans. Studies of a thoroughbred horse named 'Twilight', published in the journal *Science* in October 2009, found that she shared unusually similar chromosomal arrangements to humans. More than half of Twilight's genes appeared on chromosomes in the same order as humans, a phenomenon known as 'conserved synteny' between species. This was an unprecedented jump from the 29% of dog genes that shared this similarity to humans.

Meanwhile, conventional medicine has made little impact on the management of autistic disorders. That doesn't mean it has no role to play. It suggests rather that future solutions may mostly lie elsewhere.

Savants

Savants are people with a developmental brain disorder who have compensated with remarkable brilliance in well-defined but narrow fields. This ability contrasts with their limited skills in other areas. Savants have unusual right-hemispheric skills in art, music, mathematics or calendar calculation. It is surmised that this is due to extraordinary compensation to damage on the left side of the brain that enables a person to hyper-focus on certain skills.

Originally, they were described as idiot savants, a pejorative term. This oxymoron was an inaccurate description, because although some savants are mentally retarded, most are not. Fifty percent have autism, and the rest a developmental disability, often due to brain disease. Moreover, although many savants have autism, very few autistic persons are savants.

Two savants in modern times have become widely known. Kim Peek's story featured in the movie *The Rain Man*. He died in December 2009 and was unusual in that he was not autistic. Peek's brain had no corpus callosum, the connecting fibres between the two sides of the brain. His brain consisted of two separate halves. He had profound motor disabilities, and was unable to operate a light switch, brush his hair or button his clothes. Yet he had a bottomless memory. He was described as 'a man with islands of remarkable abilities, in a sea of disabilities'. He memorized telephone directories, and thousands of books word for word. He could read two pages in about ten seconds, the right page with his right eye, and simultaneously the left page with his left eye. He could recall details of roads on maps, and could recognize thousands of pieces of music, naming the composer and the circumstances surrounding its composition.

In a German documentary, his memory was tested by a group of American students. Their teacher tells him she was born on 5 August 1947. 'It was a Tuesday,' Kim replies, 'And this year it is a Friday. And you retire in 2012 on a Sunday.' Someone asks the name of the Oscar-winning movie when the teacher was 15 years old, 'Lawrence of Arabia,' he replies. 'That's right,' says the teacher. Peek was unique among savants. Most have a skill in a single field such as calendar calculation, music or mathematics. In comparison, Peek could master almost anything.

The other remarkable savant is Daniel Tammet. He is a brilliant high-functioning autistic savant, with remarkable mathematical ability. Tammet has contributed enormously to our understanding of the condition, because of his linguistic facility. In spite of his condition, he has been able to describe his innermost thoughts and feelings, first in his memoir *Born on a Blue Day*, and latterly in his book *Embracing the Wide Sky*.

Tammet had epilepsy and Asperger syndrome as a child. Synaesthesia is also part of his symptom complex. It involves viewing numbers as colours or sensations. He can see each integer up to 10,000 in its own unique colour, shade, texture, shape and feel. He describes for instance the number 333 as attractive and 289 as ugly. Pi is beautiful and he can recite it to its 22,514th decimal place.

Tammet is critical of Oliver Sacks' 1985 book *The Man Who Mistook His Wife for a Hat*, saying that this is a misleading portrayal of savants.

Stephen Wiltshire deserves mention. Stephen was born in London in 1974, of West Indian parents. He was mute at the age of three, and didn't learn to speak until he was nine. Yet he has the ability to sketch city landscapes from memory, having seen them just once. Stephen has drawn New York, Jerusalem, Madrid, Hong Kong, Tokyo, and many other cities in minute detail. His work has been exhibited widely, and one of his books became a *Sunday Times* bestseller.

Savants may be more common than previously recognized. Two remarkable musical savants have been studied in recent years. They are Rex Lewis-Clack in California and Derek Paravicini in England. Both are piano virtuosos and are severely disabled. Rex was born with a large cerebral cyst and, as I write, is still a teenager. Derek is now an adult. He was born 14 weeks prematurely, had to be resuscitated several times and was left blind and autistic. Yet he can play any melody from memory, and has performed with The Royal Philharmonic Orchestra, and at Ronnie Scott's Jazz Club, Buckingham Palace and Las Vegas. It is thought that his premature birth led his brain to develop separate neurological pathways, leaving him with a mixture of disability and brilliance. His capacity to memorize any musical composition simply by listening to it was gained at the expense of cutting off those neurons involved in performing everyday tasks.

The story of Rex Lewis-Clack is identical. Blind and autistic, he is also a musical savant. Both Rex and Derek have little insight and are unable to plan ahead. Kim Peek, on the other hand, had insight and was aware of his intractable motor disabilities. He said, 'You don't have to be handicapped to be different. Everyone is different,' he would tell his audiences. Tammet adds that everyone is born with certain talents, which hard work and dedication can realize. The Australian academic Professor Allan Snyder, agrees. He believes that shutting off the conscious part of the brain can unleash creativity. He claims that, in theory, we all have the innate ability to acquire some of the skills of savants. Presumably we need to rearrange the wiring of our neurons to release this intellectual energy.

Synaesthesia

The American concert pianist Laura Rosser has synaesthesia.[3] When she performs, she hears more than sounds. She hears colours. Each note has its own hue. Several famous musicians have had this rare neurological condition, including Liszt, Scriabin and Rimsky-Korsakov. And also the jazz musician Duke Ellington, who wrote *Mood Indigo*.

Synaesthesia is an unusual condition. Stimulation of one sense produces the sensation of another. Not everyone with the condition perceives sounds as colours. Some like Daniel Tammet associate colours with letters and numbers.

Synaesthesia is not a disease. On the contrary, many consider it an asset. Laura Rosser says one of her great fears as a musician is that one day she will somehow lose the ability to hear colour!

Dyslexia

Dyslexia is a disorder concerned with reading, writing and spelling. People with dyslexia may sometimes be considered backward as children, but they are not mentally retarded. Indeed, they may be highly intelligent.

The condition appears to be due to spatial difficulty with words. Dr Ian Grant-Whyte of Scottsdale, Arizona describes how as a left-handed child he was forced to become right-handed, and would mirror write words and numbers backward. He only learnt to read at the age of 40, by taking speed-reading lessons in Montreal. He used his forefinger as a pacer below the words, to prevent his eyes returning to the previous word. As an undergraduate at Cambridge University, he read the textbooks, one word at a time, and recorded the images in his brain. His ability to recall these images in examinations resembled the technique of savants.

Some believe that the extent of dyslexia has been exaggerated.[4] Graham Stringer, the Scottish Labour politician, caused outrage in 2009, by claiming that dyslexia is 'a cruel fiction'. He said it was 'time the dyslexia industry was killed off', and deplored the 'extra time dyslexics were given to complete examinations'. He added that it was absurd that a medical student should attempt to sue the General Medical Council because she was discriminated against by having to do written examinations. Stringer says, 'I want my doctors, and for that matter, dentists, engineers, teachers, and police officers, to be able to read and write.'

Professor Julian Elliott, an educational psychologist in Durham, added, 'the mushrooming of the dyslexia industry has been dramatic.' He said that it is difficult to diagnose or even define the condition, adding that 'the idea that one in ten has dyslexia is nonsense, but the issue is we are talking about so many conditions and it just keeps getting broader and broader'. The government spends almost £80 million each year on helping children with the condition. Some parents complain that many children with alleged dyslexia are gaining an unfair advantage over their classmates by claiming extra time in examinations. Indeed, there has been a 34% increase in requests for extra time, and some parents have booked private appointments to have their children diagnosed as dyslexic.

Professor John Stein of Oxford, Chairman of the Dyslexia Research Trust, says Graham Stringer is 'talking rubbish'. Nonetheless, he said it was a scandal that so many children struggled to have their learning difficulties identified.

The medical profession has largely stayed out of the debate. It is generally agreed that dyslexia is not a disease requiring medical intervention. Rather, it is an educational problem, and those with the disability require appropriate help, in the same way as people who have astigmatism or dwarfism or are colour-blind.

Quentin Tarantino

The film director Quentin Tarantino allegedly had dyslexia as a child.[5] He was hyperactive, with an IQ of 160, but had a poor performance record at school. Interviewed in 2009, by Kevin Maher for *The Times*,[6] about his latest film, Tarantino displayed residual evidence of his early problems. Maher noted that, 'despite the self-important bluster, there was insecurity and vulnerability here'. When Tarantino got excited, he mixed up his words. 'Defectors' became 'detractors', and 'offence' became 'defence'. Moreover, he could not pronounce some words at all, halting completely on 'sacrosanct'. Maher said these were 'all echoes from childhood dyslexia'. My own view is that you don't have to have dyslexia to have similar verbal difficulties from time to time!

Nonetheless Tarantino entitled his 2009 film *Inglourious Basterds*, deliberately misspelling the name. He seems to be making a statement, 'I have dyslexia and I make the rules.' Well, James Joyce challenged conventional prose, with his stream-of-consciousness style, devoid of punctuation. So far as I know, no one ever said Joyce had dyslexia.

Mental illness

Mental illness is in a different category. It covers a wide range of conditions, from eating disorders and anxiety states to mood disorders and the thought disorders or psychoses. The causes of these conditions are poorly understood in conventional pathological terms. Apart from organic illness, such as tertiary syphilis, where the spirochaete can attack the brain, causing general paralysis of the insane (GPI), we have little idea of the aetiology of mental illness. Post-mortem studies and non-invasive imaging techniques have not been helpful. Although we know a good deal about the physiology and function of the pancreas, we only have a rudimentary knowledge of the working of the mind.

For these reasons, diagnosing mental illness can sometimes be difficult. It usually involves an interview with the patient and an assessment of the psychosocial background. Psychiatrists have developed criteria for diagnosing certain conditions, but some clinical psychologists avoid diagnostic labels, preferring other methods of assessment.

The treatment of mental illness is far from satisfactory. Both medical and non-medical practitioners have been involved. There is no general agreement on therapy. It ranges from psychoanalysis and the talking doctors to those who use medication and other measures. Personality, emotional and eating disorders are often treated by psychotherapy. The psychoses are mainly the province of psychiatry, although again cognitive and behaviour therapies have their advocates.

The majority of patients with schizophrenia require medication from time to time. Unfortunately, the side effects of the medication can induce drowsiness and blunt the patient's outlook on life. Compliance is thus a problem leading to relapse. Bipolar disorders usually require mood stabilizers, and anxiety states may need anxiolytics. Although many depressed patients can be managed successfully through acute phases of their illness, many remain prone to risk of suicide.

Sadly, there have been several scandals involving the misuse of pharmacological products (see discussion elsewhere in this book). The vast majority of psychiatrists deplore this abuse of trust. Treating mental illness remains one of the greatest challenges in medicine today, and those involved have the difficult task of managing these disturbed patients in the present state of knowledge.

Richard Bentall, a clinical psychologist, is a noted opponent of orthodox psychiatry.[7] He argues, for instance, that recovery from mental illness is better in the Third World. Bentall has certainly highlighted the primitive state of the specialty, but whether his contribution to the discussion has been helpful is arguable. Another psychologist, Irving Kirsch, believes cognitive behavioural therapy is more effective than antidepressants in mood disorders. Again, many psychiatrists disagree.

Concern has been expressed by some psychiatrists in Britain that the desire not to stigmatize people has been damaging by implying there is no such thing as mental illness. In the UK, patients are now called 'service users'. In a letter to the *British Journal of Psychiatry*, 36 signatories complained that the attempt to devalue the medical model and avoid medicalization is at best confusing, and at worst damaging and even life-threatening.[8] Patients with symptoms are being referred to multidisciplinary teams, and treatment is often little more than 'jollying people along'.[9] There is no guarantee that a patient will even see a psychiatrist, and may only be prescribed psychosocial support.

It is difficult to predict the future approach to mental illness. In some respects, psychiatry is still in a formative phase – the equivalent of the 19th century approach to organic disease. Much will depend on elucidating the underlying causes of mental illness. The fact that schizophrenia-like illness can be mimicked by the use of illicit drugs suggests that there may be a biochemical basis for some of these conditions. There is also some preliminary evidence from animal experiments that there may be a molecular basis to some psychiatric disorders. Dr Mario Capecchi, a Nobel Prize-winning geneticist at the University of Utah, has shown how a group of *Hoxb8*-mutant mice, with obsessive–compulsive disorder (OCD), could be cured with a bone marrow transplant.[10] Capecchi noted that other psychiatric conditions, including depression, schizophrenia and autism, are often associated with the immune system. He believes that the experiments suggest that an immune approach to mental illness deserves further study.

In Sweden, Professor Fredrik Ullén of the Karolinska Institute has examined the density of dopamine D2 receptor genes in the thalamus together with brain scans, to study divergent thought processes. He found correlations with mental illness. The thalamus acts as a relay centre in the brain that filters information. Ullén found that people with fewer D2 receptors had less filtering and more uncensored thought. They could suspend disbelief, see unusual connections and make novel associations. They were unconstrained, with no conventional limitations and were prepared to believe anything. Among others, he quotes Salvador Dali as a man who saw the world differently, and behaved in a way that many perceived as odd. Ullén notes that creative people are uncomfortable, and it is their dissatisfaction

Biopics

Two well-known patients with schizophrenia have been the subjects of biographies and films. Their life stories have helped to bring mental illness out of the closet.

David Helfgott is an Australian concert pianist with a schizoaffective disorder. He was a child prodigy and began playing the piano at the age of five. Helfgott won a scholarship to The Royal College of Music in London, but was handicapped, if one can still use that word, by the signs and symptoms of his mental illness, which became progressively worse. At one stage, he was institutionalized and treated with electroconvulsive therapy. Nonetheless, Helfgott went on to become a well-known figure on the concert platform, and completed several world tours. His life story came to prominence in the Oscar winning film *Shine*. The similarity between the stories of David Helfgott and the musical savant Derek Paravicini is striking. It raises the question of a putative association between disability, psychosis and genius.

The second personality with schizophrenia is the American mathematician John Forbes Nash. He began his career at Princeton, working on game theory, which has applications in many areas, including computing and artificial intelligence, as well as economics. Nash's contribution to market economics led to his share of the Nobel Prize in 1994. All this was accomplished in spite of being incapacitated with paranoid delusions. His life story was portrayed in a biography written by Sylvia Nasar, later made into a film *A Beautiful Mind*.

At one stage, Nash was in and out of hospital for nearly ten years, requiring medication and insulin shock therapy. He later refused medication and said the adverse effects of these drugs are not given enough consideration. His insight into his illness is remarkable. He added that the screen depiction of him taking the newer medications was fabricated by the screenwriter, whose mother was a psychiatrist, and who was worried about encouraging patients to stop taking their drugs. Some have said the fabrication obscures an important question – whether recovery can be delayed by these drugs. It illustrates the dilemma facing psychiatrists confronted with the problem of controlling acute psychotic episodes, and the bizarre behaviour of some disturbed patients.

Nash's condition gradually improved when he led a quieter life. He speculated that his delusional status may have contributed to his creativity. He said, 'I would not have had good scientific ideas if I had thought normally.' Nash has also said that he does not see a distinction between schizophrenia and bipolar disease.

The stories of Helfgott and Nash have helped to remove some of the stigma surrounding mental illness. Both men have shown that patients with schizophrenia can sometimes function relatively normally and contribute to society, in spite of their underlying condition. One might even wonder if their exceptional contribution was *because* of their condition. Brain scans have shown similarities in the thought pathways of creative people and schizophrenics. Creative people are not constrained by the rules. They can suspend disbelief and see the world differently. They are able to 'think outside the box'.

that drives them to make changes. There is a continuum between creativity and those with psychotic traits.[11]

The current demand for evidence-based medicine indicates that the future of psychiatry will be determined by scientific findings. A biological basis is beginning to emerge from research. At the moment, it is anyone's guess where this will lead. One would like to think that there is a molecular basis for these problems, but solutions may lie elsewhere.[12]

Rewiring the cerebral cortex seems a distant goal at present. Perhaps psychiatry will move away from the medical model, and involve an amalgam of modalities, combining sociology, psychology, pharmacology and biotechnology, with artificial intelligence and nanomedicine all being involved. A hybrid specialty may emerge, a dentist of the mind.

References

1. Griffiths S. Riding to the rescue. *The Sunday Times*, 19 July 2009.
2. Wade CM, Giulotto E, Sigurdsson S et al. Genome sequence, comparative analysis, and population genetics of the domestic horse. *Science* 2009; **326**: 865–7.
3. Hamilton J. For pianist, Music unlocked rainbows of color. *National Public Radio (NPR)*, 18 April 2005.
4. Watt H. Briefing: Dyslexia. *The Sunday Times*, 18 January 2009.
5. Gilbey R. Profile: Quentin Tarantino. *The Observer*, 3 May 2009.
6. Maher K. Tarantino. Happy and inglorious. *Times 2*, 14 August 2009.
7. Bentall R. *Doctoring the Mind. Why Psychiatric Treatments Fail*. Allen Lane/Penguin: Harmondsworth, 2009.
8. Craddock N, Antebi D, Attenburrow MJ et al. Wake-up call for British psychiatry. *British Journal of Psychiatry* 2008; **193**: 6–9.
9. Hawkes N. Mentally ill are 'jollied along', rather than treated by a psychiatrist. *The Times*, 27 June 2008.
10. Chen SK, Tvrdik P, Peden E et al. Hematopoietic origin of pathological grooming in *Hoxb8* mutant mice. *Cell* 2010; **141**: 775–85.
11. Roberts M. Creative minds 'mimic schizophrenia'. *BBC News*, 29 May 2010.
12. Kirsch I. *The Emperor's New Drugs: Exploding the Antidepressant Myth*. The Bodley Head: London, 2009.

CHAPTER 11

Clinical medicine

Symptoms and signs

Before clinical medicine is consigned to the history of medicine, it is worth considering the information that can be gleaned directly from the patient. This involves listening to the patient, followed by a physical examination. Eliciting the symptoms and signs from the so-called client may even lead to a diagnosis straight away.

A careful clinical history can be extremely informative: nausea, breathlessness, palpitations, headache, urinary frequency, or bleeding from whatever site. All of these various symptoms can be distilled into a differential diagnosis, to be refined by the physical examination. The cardinal features of the clinical examination then involve four steps: inspection, palpation, percussion and auscultation.

Chapter summary

- Symptoms and signs
- The changing face of clinical medicine
- The 'Wolf wolf' syndrome
- The return of clinical medicine
- The rigours of treatment
- Cancer angst
- Awareness
- Hype, hope and expectations
- e-health and the silicon chip
- Telemedicine

Inspection

Looking at the patient is arguably the most important of the four steps. A glance can immediately reveal distress, obesity, or ill-fitting clothes and weight loss. Even the untrained eye can detect colour changes. Jaundice may suggest liver or bile duct problems, and cyanosis (blue colour) a cardiac abnormality; and a pale anaemic patient may have blood loss. The neck veins may be engorged owing to raised jugular venous pressure, suggesting heart failure. This finding may be endorsed by ankle swelling. The tips of the fingers may resemble drumsticks, a sign known to Hippocrates, now called finger clubbing. It suggests underlying lung disease. Today, finger clubbing plus nicotine staining strongly implies lung cancer. A subtle change in the facial pigmentation of young women, known as cholasma, is sometimes called the mask of pregnancy. Curious tiny blood vessel changes in the skin, called spider naevi, may imply liver cirrhosis. Again, facial weakness, ptosis (drooping eyelids), pupil changes in the eyes or an unusual gait auger neurological disorders. And a mask-like face accompanied by a tremor is a well-known 'give away' for Parkinson's disease.

Palpation

The laying on of hands is critical in cancer medicine. It can reveal splenic or liver enlargement and can detect lymph node involvement in the neck, axillae or groins. Lumps and bumps may vary in size, shape, consistency or fixation from simple lipomas to breast cancer. In cardiovascular disease, the physician can detect atrial fibrillation in the pulse at the wrist, or cardiac enlargement by feeling for the apex beat of the heart.

Then there are the intimate and sensitive examinations of the rectum and vagina. Patients do not always realize that the doctor is often as reluctant to perform a digital examination of the pelvis as the patient is to undergo it. Hence the medical dictum: 'If you fail to put your finger in it, you may put your foot in it.'

Percussion

Percussion is a more limited manoeuvre, but tapping the chest wall with one's fingers, and listening to the muffled sound, can detect a pleural effusion. Moreover, by changing the patient's position, and percussing the abdomen, one can uncover a sign known as 'shifting dullness'. It is pathognomonic of ascites or fluid in the peritoneal cavity.

Auscultation

The stethoscope is the doctor's badge of recognition. Listening for bruits, heart murmurs or adventitia in the lung fields can lead to prompt diagnosis in many cases. Then there are all the other aids to clinical diagnosis, especially in the central nervous system: the patella hammer, the tuning fork and the hatpin.

This partial list of physical signs gives only a small indication of the information that can be deduced from a thorough physical examination. Comprehensive lists of the symptoms and signs of a multitude of disorders have filled many distinguished textbooks.

Beyond these lists, there are extended examples of the role of clinical medicine in certain specialties. In gynaecology for instance, a fairly clear idea of the diagnosis can often be gained simply from taking a careful *history* from the patient. In paediatric cardiology, an indication of the cardiac status of a child can sometimes be obtained from *palpation* alone, without even the use of the stethoscope. Above all, there is one specialty that relies crucially on *inspection*, namely dermatology.

The changing face of clinical medicine

Some years ago, Alice Trillin, a New York schoolteacher, wrote an article in the *New England Journal of Medicine* entitled 'Of Dragons and Garden Peas'. In it, she described her experience as a patient. She said that doctors and patients are accomplices in acting out a kind of drama. Doctors defy death. That is what they are trained to do. She said that for a patient it immediately becomes clear that the best thing you can do to please your doctor is to be healthy. If you can't do that, the next best thing is to be well behaved (see Chapter 24).

Is this true today? Certainly patients are better informed. The Internet has replaced the *Reader's Digest*. And physicians are more open in discussing treatment and outcome. However, there is a more disturbing trend: the demise of the physical examination. It has been derided as 'poking and prodding'. One critical author tells how, as a heart patient, he went to see his physician. And the doctor got out a rubber hammer and banged it on his knee. The same writer failed to mention, or notice, whether the doctor also used the stethoscope, or apply the above four cardinal clinical steps: all of which can reveal cardiac status on the spot. There are, incidentally, several reasons why a cardiac physician might check the central nervous system with a patella hammer. They include checking for emboli from atrial fibrillation.

Professor Joe Connon from Toronto described how, as a visiting professor in California, he presided over Grand Rounds (a pretentious term). Connon said that the clinical history, examination and physical findings were presented in a couple of minutes, and the rest of the hour was devoted entirely to the investigations and discussion.

I can expand on that. When I was winding down my post overseas, I overlapped with my replacement, who was an intelligent physician. We saw a patient together at follow-up. She had a past history of a subungual melanoma under the left thumbnail. She now complained of dyspnoea – breathlessness. Without examining the patient, my new colleague set about ordering a battery of tests, blood work, X-rays and scans.

Already from a glance at the patient, I could see that she looked gravely ill (*inspection*). I put a hand in her axilla and felt a hard fixed lump the size of a golfball (*palpation*). Her chest was stony dull (*percussion*), evidence of a pleural effusion. It wasn't even necessary to take the stethoscope out of the bag (*auscultation*). Sadly, the patient had pathognomonic signs of widespread metastases. The observation took about two minutes. This was not advanced clinical medicine. It is a requirement of the final medical degree examination, pass or fail.

The medical training programme has been revamped so often that it seems unable to achieve a balance. A prominent College President told me about the final-year medical student who knew all about handling bereavement, but knew nothing about the causes. A senior colleague in Boston used to say he would prefer to be seen by an older physician, rather than a younger doctor who might be overly influenced by an article in last week's *New England Journal of Medicine*.

Patients carry some responsibility. Often they don't want to be examined. They want an MRI. Moreover, reports of new discoveries and breakthroughs have increased demands for the latest advance, frequently before it has been fully tested. It can be summed up in a piece of doggerel:

> *Patients decline*
> *Symptom and sign,*
> *Preferring instead*
> *Tests, it is said.*

Sometimes the doctor is happy to offload the responsibility to technology for several reasons. First, it is easier and faster, especially if his or her clinical skills are diminishing. Second, it keeps the patient happy. Third, it provides some degree of cover against litigation.

A similar situation has been evident in prescribing treatment. It is quicker to write a script than to spend time discussing the problem. For, in the end, the patient usually expects the compulsory piece of paper.

It is clear where this is heading. The physician has abrogated responsibility. The nurse assistant can do the job, order the test(s) and, as we shall see, occasionally interpret the results, and even prescribe the treatment.

The 'Wolf wolf' syndrome

In the debate between the art and the science of medicine, science wins hands down. Sadly, like the skills of any ancient craft, the art may soon be lost completely.

I have an example of this. Towards the latter half of my career, especially during my time overseas, I would see many patients at cancer follow-up visits. When a patient that I knew well came through the door, I could often tell immediately, by their demeanour, whether they were ill. My wife calls this gravitas.

But this ability to distinguish the sick from the walking well is not confined to doctors. Friends can often tell at a glance whether their 'buddies are in good shape'. 'My, you are looking well' is a common greeting among the retired community.

The art of medicine may also involve clinical acumen. In eliciting a follow-up history, patients may communicate in their own vernacular. In Northern Ireland, when they are symptom-free, they might say, 'I'm bravely doctor.' In Bermuda, if unwell, they might say, 'I have bad feelings.' Interpreting this can involve more than language. Gestures and facial expression may be helpful. Probing may uncover a nuance, an occasional headache, a loss of interest, or appetite or energy, but nothing specific. Physical examination and tests may be normal.

Other patients may be more forthcoming: a list of symptoms, sometimes transient, sometimes persistent. The patient may arrive with a written list of miscellaneous events. Again, examination reveals no abnormal signs, and investigations are negative. But lethargy and symptoms persist, over a year or longer. The physician may even be tempted to label the patient a hypochondriac. Not in my view, if there is a history of cancer.

Too often have I seen the sinister findings emerge after several years of fruitless investigations. The abnormalities have been below the threshold of measurement.

But the human protoplasm knew all along that there were rogue molecules in the system. I have called this clinical condition the 'Wolf wolf syndrome'. Beware of the patient who cries, 'Wolf, wolf!'

It may be that we will eventually have a molecular handle on this set of symptoms. For the moment, the art survives, although it remains under threat. Changes are on the way.

The return of clinical medicine

Fortunately there is some evidence of a possible return to clinical medicine, albeit not widely known. A study in the *BMJ* from the London Chest Hospital followed 8176 patients who presented with chest pain or suspected angina. Angina is the most common symptom of heart disease. The standard practice is to refer the patient to a rapid-access clinic for an electrocardiograph (ECG) to decide whether additional attention is required. Those with cardiac abnormalities then receive appropriate treatment. Patients with normal ECGs are often further assessed with a stress test, i.e. an exercise ECG.

The study then followed the outcome of all patients, 60% of whom had had a stress test. Over the subsequent few years, almost 50% of all coronary 'events', such as heart attacks, occurred in patients whose ECGs were normal. It was found that routine clinical assessment, which involved taking a detailed history and a thorough physical examination, was almost as good as a stress test in predicting future heart disease.

It was concluded that tests are of limited value and no substitute for quizzing patients and examining them.[1] This is of course time-consuming. It involves listening to patients. 'Communication skills' is the buzz term.

The clinical examination of patients has not completely disappeared. David Jones, the boss of Next, the £3.5 billion high-street retail store, describes in his autobiography how, at the age of 39, he went for a routine company medical check-up. Jones says, 'during the physical examination, the doctor stopped writing his notes. He took off my glasses and gently tapped my forehead just above the bridge of my nose. "You've got Parkinson's disease", he said.' The eye blink test had confirmed the diagnosis, without the need for investigations of any kind.

There is another clinical area where the machine cannot go. That is in the indistinct boundary between a nuisance and an illness.[3] Dr Lennard-Jones, a London physician, noted that this is often apparent in gastrointestinal disorders. He states, 'There is no dividing line between health and disease, only between those who shrug off their symptoms, seeking little or no medical help, and those whose lives are affected to a greater or lesser extent by a troublesome gastrointestinal tract.' In this borderland zone, it is not the illness that matters, but how you handle that illness. In this area the machine has no role.

The rigours of treatment

Medicine has been evolving throughout history. The increasing reliance on investigations is a relatively recent phenomenon. It isn't that long ago that we were in the dark ages. I have earlier outlined the graphic description of the multifarious and useless treatments forced down the mouth of the dying King Charles II by the dozen or so royal physicians of the day. The catalogue of nostrums, herbs and poisons prescribed makes one wonder how the medical profession survived with any credibility at all.

And what will the future make of the recent past in my own specialty, oncology: the mutilating radical Halstead mastectomy, radiation fibrosis, massive lymphoedema, alopecia, nausea, neutropenia and neuropathy. Or worse, 'chemo-brain' (chemotherapy-induced cognitive decline).

Not long ago, a teenage girl in Glasgow with advanced leukaemia said 'enough' and declined further treatment. Her courage in defeat was commended and made headlines.[4] An even younger 13-year-old girl, Hannah Jones, who had previously had leukaemia, won a legal battle against an attempt to force her to have a heart transplant against her wishes. She said she wanted to die with dignity, but child protection officers were called in, and threatened to remove her from her parents' custody to make her have surgery.

The management of advanced incurable disease is a minefield for oncologists. The most difficult decision for any doctor is when not to treat. How much more difficult again for the patient to receive the news. A former US Presidential candidate, Senator Hubert Humphrey, famously described his chemotherapy as 'bottled death'. One distinguished physician in Boston told me her father blew his brains out, rather than continue with treatment for bladder cancer. Most patients of course accept the rigours of treatment. It beats the alternative. And, besides, the amelioration of side effects has improved.

Cancer angst

Breaking the news

As we move inexorably into the age of technology, clinical contact with patients is being eroded. There remains one area, however, where the physician cannot avoid making contact with the patient. That is in conveying bad news.

Breaking the news of a cancer diagnosis has always been difficult. In 1873, Thomas Percival wrote in *Medical Ethics* that 'to a patient … who makes inquiries which, if faithfully answered, might prove fatal to him, it would be a gross and unfeeling wrong to tell the truth'. The argument whether to tell the whole truth to every patient – always assuming the doctor knows the truth – has been debated for many years. Today, breaking the news is not any easier, but there are two important differences. First, in the 19th century, there were no cures. Today, many malignancies are curable, and most are amenable to some form of treatment, if only palliative. Second, there is now the legal requirement of informed consent, although this sometimes only applies if some form of intervention is planned.

Most doctors today tell the patient 'up front'. Some make a clumsy attempt at breaking the news, others have been accused of being cold and indifferent. Part of the doctor's problem has been attributed to facing up to his own mortality. Part of the patient's problem is 'shooting the messenger'. Criticism of the doctor's communication skills is often warranted, but there is no way of making bad news, good news. The main features of communication remain sincerity, honesty and compassion.

A young medical student, John McCool, with a brain tumour, wrote to me many years ago as follows:[5]

> *A lot of people these days mourn the passing of the old time family doctor, the family friend, always available, and always ready to listen and dispense advice. They decry contemporary high tech medicine for its loss of intimacy and warmth, and for the increasing distance between doctor and patient. Yet who would argue that today's medicine is not infinitely preferable to old time medicine, impotent and largely ignorant, for all its warmth of reassurance. For in the end, to paraphrase Lewis Thomas, if I develop a brain tumour, I want as much comfort and friendship as are available, but mainly I want quick and effective treatment so that I may, if that is possible, survive.*

In fairness, providing effective treatment and having a sympathetic manner are not mutually exclusive. It is possible to have both.

The strain on the doctor on telling the patient is always present. Dr Saul Radovosky relates how, early in his career, a patient in Boston, who wanted to be told everything, when told everything went on 'shrieking and tearing at herself for days, unnerving her sick neighbours, and deeply affecting me'.[6]

Dr Tony Calland relates the harrowing moment he had to break the news of lung cancer to his best friend and tennis partner.[7] He called at his friend's home inadvertently at a happy family tea party, 'knowing that in a few minutes I would utter the words that would set in motion a train of events that would mean that that family would never be the same again. I decided general practice had its drawbacks'. When his friend died, Calland said, 'I have never felt as I did then. I felt that I had failed him, not because he had suffered or been in pain, but because I was his friend, and I was his doctor, and the science of medicine had not made him better.'

John Betjeman captures the sombre mood on receiving the diagnosis in his poem Devonshire Street W1 (see box).

On a lighter note, the actress Sheila Hancock relates the ludicrous pantomime when she tried to obtain the truth about her mother's diagnosis.[8] Following the laparotomy, Sheila asked the nurse what they had found: 'She said, "You must ask the sister", who said I must ask the doctor, who said I must ask the surgeon who performed the operation.'

After some days, Sheila was back in the hospital when the surgeon was doing his rounds. He was a caricature of Sir Lancelot Spratt, straight out of Richard Gordon's classic tale *Doctor in the House*:

"No star of the stage has ever been treated like that man. Before he arrived, nurses were flying around tidying away flowers and books, making beds, pushing patients into them, washing them and combing their hair. 'You want to look nice for the doctor, don't you?' Sister was more nervous than any theatre director I have seen on a first night. The atmosphere was electric".

Then in burst the great man himself, surrounded by his minions. He addressed an occasional word to the specimens, but most of the chat was to the students

Devonshire Street W1

Poem by John Betjeman

The heavy mahogany door with its wrought-iron screen
Shuts. And the sound is rich, sympathetic, discreet.
The sun still shines on this eighteenth-century scene
With Edwardian faience adornment – Devonshire Street.

No hope. And the X-ray photographs under his arm
Confirm the message. His wife stands timidly by.
The opposite brick-built house looks lofty and calm
Its chimneys steady against the mackerel sky.

No hope. And the iron knob of this palisade
So cold to the touch, is luckier now than he
'Oh merciless, hurrying Londoners! Why was I made
For the long and painful deathbed coming to me?'

She puts her fingers in his, as, loving and silly
At long-past Kensington dances she used to do
'It's cheaper to take the tube to Piccadilly
And then we can catch a nineteen or twenty-two.'

Reproduced by permission of John Murray (Publishers) Limited.

and that in an unintelligible mutter. He seemed unable actually to look a patient straight in the eyes, presumably preferring the sight of their surgical scars.

Sheila adds graciously that not all surgeons are like that. But on this occasion it was impossible to hold up the royal procession with banal questions like 'What have you done, or are going to do to me?' And certainly not 'Am I dying?'

Although Sheila Hancock deplores much of the way the medical information is handled and transmitted, she fully appreciates the problems involved. She agrees that doctors and nurses have real problems in facing the inevitability of their own deaths. She adds that 'interestingly my overwhelming feeling later, on meeting the consultant, was pity for that man having to tell me the news. He was by nature and training so bad at communication, I felt that whatever happened, I shouldn't embarrass him by showing distress.'

Living with the news

Elsewhere, I have described the feelings of the Irish author Nuala O'Faolain on learning she had cancer: 'Life had lost its beauty.'

In another instance, a young patient of mine, Campbell Moreland, a 29-year-old doctor with cancer, wrote of his experience in *The Lancet*.[9] He likened it to solitary confinement:

Once inside the prison cell you are trapped; you can walk around, examine the furniture, scrutinise the walls until you know every crack in the plaster, and look out the window; sometimes the door will open and fresh air will enter; yet it is impossible to step over the line dividing the cell from the corridor. The most useful people and the best doctors are those prepared to come inside the cell, sit down and spend some time with you. The outsider can then adjust his or her horizon to that of the patient, and will be able to see the cell much as the patient sees it, although never quite the same. A person of no help to the patient is the one who opens the hatch and says, 'I can see your cell, its furniture, the cracks in the wall, but I am not coming in. Here are some books, have an injection, things will soon be all right, and you will be able to come out', closes the hatch and disappears.

Some years earlier, Ron Klingbeil, a 13-year-old boy with cancer in Michigan expressed similar feelings:[10]

Fear is today and dying now. You slip in and out of my room, give me medication, and check my blood pressure. Is it because you are insecure, don't know what to say, don't know what to do? I am the one who is dying. Don't run away. Wait. Death may get to be a routine to you, but it is new to me.

Barbara Ehrenreich, the author, feminist and political activist, was diagnosed with breast cancer. She wrote of her experience in *Harper's Magazine* and the London *Times*.[11] When she was diagnosed, she found the disease had been hijacked by a culture of celebrity and sentiment. She said women confronting a life-threatening illness deserve better than teddy bears and angel pins.

She tells how a routine mammogram gave rise to some 'concern' and had to be repeated. So she came back, waiting for the result in the role of suspect, eager to clear her name. Then, following a biopsy, the physician said, 'Unfortunately there is a cancer.' She adds, 'the most heinous thing about that remark was not the presence of cancer, but the absence of me. Where I once was a person, I was now a "cancer".' She relates that from then on the career of a breast cancer patient is pretty well mapped out. You might get to negotiate the treatment a little, but you are now part of the system. Ehrenreich deplores the cult of the pink ribbon and the mindless triumphalism of 'survivorhood'. She asks, 'Did we who live, fight harder than those who died? Can we claim to be braver, better people than the dead?' She found that cheerfulness is mandatory, and dissent a kind of treason. 'Why', she concludes, 'is there no room for some gracious acceptance of death, when the time comes, which it surely will, through cancer or other misfortune?'

These thoughts on terminal illness are not confined to cancer. Arthur Ashe, the tennis champion, contracted AIDS through a blood transfusion. When he was dying, he wrote a book dedicated to his daughter entitled *Days of Grace*. It was a moving acceptance of his fate. He was 49 years old when he died.

There are other fatal conditions. One Saturday morning some time ago, my wife and daughter by chance met a close friend of mine. His voice was slurred. Stan enjoyed a glass of wine, but not in the morning. Only later did we realize he had bulbar palsy, an early symptom of motor neuron disease. In time, his condition deteriorated and his son returned home from Scotland for a visit. Stan was upset and having difficulty getting dressed. His wife said, 'Relax Stan. Take it easy.'

'I can't', he replied, 'I have never died before.' Stan stared his fate straight in the face and died the next day.

This confrontation between life and death is not the prerogative of medicine. It is part of the human condition.

Awareness

There is another area where the art and science of medicine overlap. That is in the level of patient awareness. The most disturbing example of this is in anaesthesia. Rarely – happily very rarely – patients may actually be awake during surgery, but unable to communicate their feelings because they are paralysed by curare-like drugs. I had one example of this some years ago in the USA. The patient told me that she had been awake while undergoing surgical resection for cancer of the oesophagus. The surgeon and anaesthesiologist did not realize that she had been awake throughout the procedure! This horror situation can still occur, albeit rarely. Anaesthetists recognize the problem, and are striving to overcome it. It is hoped that scientific advances will soon be able to detect the level of patient awareness during surgery.

It is not only under anaesthesia that patients may be conscious of their surroundings, yet unable to communicate their feelings. Students and young doctors have been taught to be careful in discussing the clinical outcome in front of patients who may seem to be asleep. From time to time, physicians forget this advice. Elsewhere, I have related the story of an unconscious patient dying of ovarian cancer, who surfaced briefly to enquire why her intravenous drip had been removed.

One of the more controversial cases of patient awareness was reported from Belgium in 2009.[12] Following a road accident, Rom Houben was allegedly locked in a coma for 23 years. During that time, it was claimed he remained fully conscious of his surroundings, but unable to communicate. His condition emerged when his carer, Linda Wouters, noted that when she spoke to him, he would waggle his toe. Eventually, she found that she was able to elicit a response by guiding his hand over a computer screen. He described his reawakening and said, 'I am blessed. Someone had thrown away the keys forever.' He added, 'In the eyes of the world, I was a sporty young man who had suddenly become a vegetable … I was there, day in, day out, I saw, I felt, but only deep inside, hidden from everyone, but not from myself.'

Many experts are now sceptical of the findings, and suggest that this was another case of 'Ouija board messages'. The name of the Ouija board – 'yes/yes board' – is derived from the French 'oui' and the German 'ja'. It is used in séances in the occult world and has mostly been discredited. It is often the observer who is doing the pointing, who is creating the messages. The technique is known as *facilitated communication*, a controversial speech-aided method that has the patient reliant on the hand of the therapist to pick out letters on a keyboard.

The doctor at the centre of the report on the Houben case, Dr Steven Laureys, is concerned that he may have been duped to some extent, but nevertheless is keen to follow up the study of awareness in semiconscious patients.[13]

Dr Martin Monty of the Medical Research Council Cognition and Brain Science Unit at Cambridge said, 'There is a difference between someone who is conscious and unable to move, and someone who is unable to move because they are unconscious.' Rom Houben's case has reopened the entire field of assessing so-called comatose patients. An extended study of 23 patients in a vegetative state used functional magnetic resonance imaging (fMRI) to detect brain activity and awareness. Four of the patients responded accurately to questions. In another study, using the Coma Recovery Scale (CRS), 18 of 44 'vegetative' patients had been misdiagnosed. There is a new awareness of awareness.

A story from the past illustrates the different functional components of the brain. The late Dr Louis Hurwitz related a tale from Queen Square Hospital, London, where he trained as a neurologist. Around the time of the Boer War in South Africa, one ward in the hospital contained a number of wounded veterans in various states of confusion. One day, a young subaltern rushed into the ward and cried out, 'Mafeking has been relieved.' With that, many of the old soldiers scrambled out of bed, stood at attention, saluted, and sang 'God save the King', then fell back in bed into their former stuperose state. Hurwitz claimed that a different part of the brain, dealing with emotional matters, reacted momentarily to the news, then spontaneously relapsed.

There is a fourth group of patients who may appear outwardly unaware of their surroundings. My brother, a former orthopaedic surgeon, tells how, some years ago, he went to see an elderly colleague confined to hospital with early dementia. My brother chatted to the patient for half an hour or so, but it was a struggle, a one-way conversation. As he was about to leave, the nurse came in and said, 'Well, I suppose your friend hardly recognized you.' At which point, the seemingly vacuous patient sat up suddenly in bed and said, 'Don't talk nonsense nurse, that's John Lowry.'

Parents of young children will not be surprised at these tales of second childhood. For it is widely recognized that infants and toddlers fully understand what is going on around them, and can point to what they want, long before they can speak.

Hype, hope and expectations

Medicine has been the victim of its own success. Because of the scientific advances from the discovery of insulin, penicillin, DNA, transplant surgery, and so on, patients have come to expect miracles. It should be a golden era. Disease should have been conquered.

If we can get to the Moon, why haven't we cured the common cold? It is a fair question and deserves a response. The answer is that the cold, like influenza, is caused by a virus. While viruses do not respond to antibiotics, vaccination is often effective. But although there are three main types of flu virus, there are hundreds of different types of cold virus.

The influenza virus changes its structure, which is why a new vaccine has to be prepared every year. A vaccine for the cold virus would be possible, but because there are so many types that are constantly mutating, a new vaccine would have to be produced every week! Again, by the time it had been developed, it would be hopelessly out of date, as the virus changes its coat and moves on. Moreover, although flu can be debilitating, the common cold is less severe, and may only last a few days. There is less incentive for funding organizations to support long-term research on this topic.

In passing, it is worth noting that there is some controversy about the effectiveness of flu vaccines.[14] Critics have suggested that the mortality difference between vaccinated and unvaccinated individuals may be due to the 'healthy user effect'. People who get vaccinated are more motivated and healthier than those who don't. The debate is unlikely to be resolved, because no one is contemplating a controlled trial with an untreated placebo arm.

The demand for a cure for every ailment has sometimes led to dissatisfaction with the local doctor. If he or she cannot cure your illness, mild or serious, go abroad for a second opinion, if you can afford it. Or try alternative medicine, even if you cannot afford it. One recalls celebrities from the past – Steve McQueen, Yul Brunner, and others – who made fruitless trips abroad seeking nostrums for incurable disease.

Many forces conspire to exaggerate success in medicine. First, there is the public desire for a breakthrough. Second, there is media hype eager to feed this demand. Third, there are the pharmaceutical companies anxious to promote their products. Less obvious are the fundraising bodies, boosting scientific progress on the one hand, yet paradoxically highlighting the continuing battle, in order to obtain financial support.

Some of this publicity has backfired. A few years ago, *Scientific American* published an article entitled 'We are losing the war against cancer'. And *Time* magazine, referring to the invincible cancers, ran a cover story, 'More hype than hope'.

Is it true today? Not quite. Cancer may not be eradicated, but there has been considerable progress, especially in molecular medicine, the understanding of disease and the development of designer drugs. Antibiotics did not eradicate bacteria, but they transformed the treatment of infectious disease. Personally, I believe success is in sight, not by Monday morning, but probably by Friday afternoon.

e-health and the silicon chip

While biology is racing ahead, leaving clinical medicine behind, developments are moving equally rapidly in the field of electronics and information technology. Computerized medicine is transforming health care. When classical physics moved from the conduction of electrons in gases to solid-state physics, the semiconductor was born. Semiconductors are intermediate between conductors and insulators; thus they can conduct electrons under some conditions, but not others. The transistor is a semiconductor device that can amplify or switch electronic signals. It is the active component of modern electronics, and can consist of a single discrete

The wages of medicine

A recent headline read 'British doctors are Europe's richest'. Both consultants and general practitioners are now better off than their colleagues in France, Germany, Denmark, Sweden, Finland and Portugal. And they earn ten times as much as doctors in the Czech Republic or Hungary. This was confirmed for me by a radiologist who attended a meeting in Prague. He met a Czech colleague who told him he flew to London at weekends to do locums, and earned more in the two days in Britain than in a month in Prague.

The problems the medical profession has with government in Britain are not entirely to do with money. Part of it may have to do with staffing. Italy for instance has twice as many doctors per thousand people than the UK.

The situation in the USA is different again. Incomes are often over a quarter of a million dollars, depending on the speciality and the practice. At the same time, malpractice premiums can be exorbitant. In some cases, an obstetrician's premium may exceed an internist's income.

Declining status

Once upon a time, physicians had prestige and standing in the community. The decline in status is a relatively recent phenomenon. There are several reasons for the attitudinal change.

Doctor no longer knows best. He or she is human and makes mistakes. This is more evident in an open society. Second, scientific advances have raised expectations to unrealistic levels. Patients are more demanding. When the doctor doesn't deliver, he is criticized, by-passed, and maybe even sued. The third change is more subtle, and often unspoken. It is envy. In uncertain economic times, the salaries of doctors, especially GPs in the UK, are sometimes considered exorbitant for what is on offer.

In an article in *The Times* in 2010 entitled 'If you must get ill, make sure it is before 6 pm', Libby Purves wrote, 'In 2004 the Government blithely signed a new contract with family doctors, boosting their pay by 30 per cent, while crucially allowing them to opt out of any responsibility for their patients outside surgery hours'.

Hospital consultants are also under fire from health service unions who claim that clinical excellence awards are excessive.

In the USA, many patients previously went bankrupt paying health bills. That may be about to change. In Britain, the medical profession has been blamed for blocking reform. A Health Minister in the UK government said that the problems of the NHS were the doctors' fault. The doctor has become a scapegoat. Even alternative practitioners have been quick to criticize, claiming most physicians ignore the patient's wider problems, the so-called holistic approach.

Some of these criticisms are fair. Most are not. The doctor may not be a fallen angel, but he sometimes appears a fractured saint. Either way, things are not what they used to be. Years ago the physician was often revered (see Figure 12.1 and Colour Plate 3: George Forbes MD).

To the Memory
of
GEORGE FORBES MD
Whom living
A singular complacency of manners
Joined with many useful talents
And eminent virtues
Render'd highly estimable
Bless'd with a convivial disposition
In the cheerful hour of social festivity
He shone irreprehensible.
An agreeable Companion,
Ever assiduous in furthering good humour
And the enjoyments of sociality
Friendly to Mankind,
His endeavors to mitigate the evils of life
Which he bore himself with temper and philosophy,
Were not alone confined to the *Healing art*,
Long exercised by him with much Reputation;
But were likewise exerted
In composing differences,
Restoring ancient friendships interrupted
And promoting
Peace, harmony, and mutual good understanding
Among his fellow men.
Having acquitted himself with approbation
In the several relations of life
As he had lived respected and beloved,
So he died
Lamented and regretted for these virtues
And many others
Which
Tho' not enregister'd on this Marble,
Are for ever engraven
On the Memory of his many sorrowing friends!
He died Jan 9th 1778 Aged 68

Figure 12.1 *George Forbes, MD: an 18th century memorial tablet to a revered physician, in St Peter's Church, Bermuda – the oldest continuously used Anglican Church in the Western Hemisphere.*

The writer and broadcaster the late Alistair Cooke was able to tell the following amusing story. It concerned the imaginary inauguration of the first Jewish President of the USA. Following the ceremony, the Chief Justice of the Supreme Court turned to the new President's mother, Mrs Ginsburg, to congratulate her. 'Ah yes', replied the elderly lady, 'but my other son, he is a doctor!'

Modernizing medicine

Many of the problems in the industrial world are concerned with modernization, pay and working conditions. Medicine has had identical problems.

A document prepared by the Department of Health in the UK in 2006,[4] entitled *Modernising Medical Careers* (MMC), resulted in turmoil among junior doctors. The then Minister of Health, Patricia Hewitt, was forced to apologize and ordered an inquiry. Sir John Tooke chaired the inquiry. His report highlighted many of the problems and made a number of recommendations, only some of which were accepted by government.

It was particularly noted there is no consensus as to where medicine is heading. The section entitled 'The Role of the Doctor' begins with the following statement:

Service needs cannot be met now or in the future, unless there is a clear understanding of what part each health care professional plays. This is particularly true for doctors and needs to be articulated ...

Without such definitions it is impracticable to pursue outcome focussed medical education, or attempt to plan the workforce ... The doctor's role as diagnostician and the handler of clinical uncertainty and ambiguity, requires a sound educational base in science and evidence based practice, as well as research awareness.

The section concludes:

There needs to be a common shared understanding of the roles of all doctors in the contemporary health care team that takes account of public expectations.

Responding to the report, Paul Streets, Chief Executive of the Postgraduate Medical Education and Training Board, said:

The report calls for a debate about the role of doctors. Without a clear widely supported view of the skills and knowledge required by doctors of the future, we run the risk of training doctors for careers which may not be relevant to future need.

Parveen Kumar, Past President of the BMA, added that the report highlighted that:

There is no consensus on the actual role of doctors for the future – vital for organizing and developing future training.

Tooke's report also:

revealed evidence that education and training opportunities for doctors were being diminished, by such experiences being used for other health care professionals substituting for medical practitioner roles. Although such skill-mix solutions may be superficially attractive to meet service performance imperatives, they call into question the clarity of role of other contributors to the health care team, and whether role 'substitutors' have the necessary educational foundations to execute the roles to the required high standards.

Although not named in the report, 'role substitutors' mainly refers to nurse consultants/specialists/practitioners. In a recent lecture, Sir John Tooke outlined several other developments that will determine the future role of the doctor. In addition to role substitution, he lists climate change, globalization and technological advances.

Planning ahead

It is difficult to plan ahead, when there is no clear view on the future of medical care (see Figure 12.2). It may perhaps be appropriate to start with the recruitment of medical students. One might look for those who have a 'calling', a vocation. But it is said that candidates have been advised that if asked at interview, 'Why do you want to study medicine?', they should never reply, 'Because I want to help people.' That is deemed naive, no longer politically correct (PC). A colleague quips, 'In that case, the only answer is, for the money!'

More seriously, Dr Marcia Angell, former Editor of the *New England Journal of Medicine*, a distinguished physician, named by *Time* magazine in 1997 as one of the 25 most influential Americans, says, 'I know it sounds trite, but I wanted to be a doctor so I could help sick people feel better. Even as a small child, I thought there was something particularly cruel about ill health – in that it struck capriciously and sometimes made it impossible to enjoy any other aspect of life.' She adds that she now works in Social and Preventive Medicine, and says, 'Thus my original desire to take care of sick people, one at a time, was never realized.'

Elsewhere, Professor John Crown relates the case of an Irish girl, who achieved top marks in her Leaving Certificate examination, but was refused entry to medical school because she failed a 'non-validated multiple-choice aptitude test'. Crown believes there is no exam that can tell us who will be a good doctor.[5]

Tooke, however, outlines several important features required of the future physician. These include clinical reasoning, the ability to synthesize information, and leadership. He notes that medicine is a risky business, and that the doctor needs to be able to manage uncertainty. Risk profiling and risk aversion will be increasingly important for patients. He cautions that even diagnostic screening is never 100% effective.

Medicine has diverged into over 50 subspecialties, and this number is increasing. At the last count, there were 57 categories. This fragmentation has been accompanied by a renewed focus on primary care, in an attempt to coordinate all this activity. The general practitioner remains the gatekeeper in the community, but in hospitals it is the nurse who is in charge of triage.

My own view is that scientific and technical advances will determine the future of the profession. The physician is gradually being replaced by the health technician and the machine. At least as significant as the changing roles of doctors are the changing expectations of patients. Doctors are increasingly being challenged. Medicine has been on the back foot. The profession has yet to come to terms with the attitudinal change, and the shift in the nature of health care. At times this may seem bewildering. Modernizing medicine calls for collaboration and cool heads.

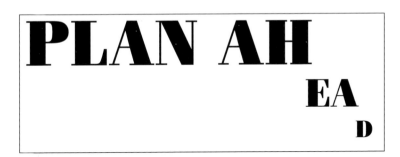

Figure 12.2 *Plan Ahead*

The three-year medical degree

More radical changes are underway in America. Increasingly, it is recognized that the lengthy medical training programme may not always be necessary. Texas Tech University is to offer the first three-year MD programmme in the USA. Students will enrol in Lubbock, Texas, starting in September 2010. The move is to encourage more doctors to enter primary care. The curriculum timetable is being reorganized to focus on family medicine. The Texas programme is called 'The Family Medicine Accelerated Track'. Experts agree that America needs more primary care physicians, rather than medical specialists.

Texas Tech announced the new plan the same day President Barak Obama signed health care reform legislation. The new Bill is expected to add millions of people to doctors' lists in 2014, when the law's major provisions take effect.

Two Canadian institutions, McMaster University and The University of Calgary, already offer three-year MD degrees, but Texas Tech is the first in the USA. This raises questions about the fourth year of most American degrees, and indeed the longer training programmes in Britain and elsewhere.

The Carnegie Endowment for Advanced Teaching is expected to recommend, among other things, that all American medical schools should consider the three-year option. David Irby, of the University of California in San Francisco, and co-director of the study, says that the coming debate is likely to be controversial. In Britain, the plan would probably cause consternation. But changes are inevitable. Medicine is moving inexorably into a new era.

Moreover, the debate has yet to take account of the new health professional, the physician assistant, merging seamlessly into the medical world. This is discussed in a later chapter.

References

1. Laurance J. The medical time bomb. Too many women doctors. *The Independent*, 2 August 2004.
2. Driscoll M. Women doctors: the waste of money you will be glad to see. *The Sunday Times*, 9 May 2010.
3. Woolcock N. Girls need lessons in juggling career and family life. *The Times*, 14 November 2009.
4. Tooke J. *Final Report of the Independent Inquiry into Modernising Medical Careers. Aspiring to Excellence*. Universities UK, London, 8 January 2008.
5. Crown J. There is no exam that can tell us who will be a good doctor. *The Sunday Independent (Ireland)*, 23 August 2009.

CHAPTER 13

Compassion

The loss of compassion

One of the casualties in the decline of medicine is the loss of compassion. Patients no longer want to be examined. They want an MRI. Gradually the physician is being replaced by the machine. The machine has no feelings, no compassion. Even the Dalai Lama has written a book on the subject. What is this elusive quality called compassion, and can it be measured? Can it be recovered? And does it matter?[1]

Compassion is a form of altruism. It involves empathy and passionate concern for the welfare of others. It has been defined as caring for others as you would wish for yourself. In medicine, it is a feeling of distress for the suffering of patients, and a desire to alleviate their misfortune.

Compassion is certainly not confined to medicine. All the great social reformers were compassionate: John Howard and penal reform, Elizabeth Fry and Newgate Prison, Shaftsbury and his Factory Act, Wilberforce and slavery. In the USA, John Quincy Adams worked tirelessly to repeal the 'Gag Act' that prevented slavery from being discussed in Congress. More recently, Albert Camus in France, in his novel *The Plague*, expressed his feelings of compassion for the victims of the epidemic of cholera in Algeria (see box).

Shakespeare documented mental torment, physical deformity and disease in many of his plays.[2] Charles Dickens had compassion in full measure.[3] He was first a novelist, but also a social reformer, and often visited hospitals and prisons. Dickens gave accurate descriptions of many physical and mental illnesses.[4] These observations included most famously the Pickwickian syndrome, the fat boy with obstructive apnoea, but he also described movement disorders, Ménière's disease and even acute leukaemia. Dickens went further and made positive suggestions. On visiting a Boston asylum, he declared that moral influence, born of kindness and caring, was more effective at controlling violent psychotic patients than straitjackets.

Walt Whitman, the leading American poet of the 19th century, expressed his concern for victims of the Civil War. As a hospital visitor, he attended thousands

The Plague

Albert Camus, the French philosopher and author, based his novel *The Plague*, on a cholera epidemic in the Algerian city of Oran. Camus' fictional physician, Dr Bernard Rieux, expresses his feelings of solidarity and compassion for the infected citizens:

In the midst of the epidemic, the plague had swallowed up everything and everyone ... the truth is nothing is less sensational than pestilence, and by reason of their very duration, great misfortunes are monotonous. Dr Rieux resolved to compile his chronicle, so that he should not be one of those who hold their peace, but should bear witness in favour of those plague-stricken people; so that some memorial of the injustice and outrage done to them might endure; and to state quite simply what we learn in time of pestilence: that there are more things to admire in men than to despise.

of severely wounded soldiers. The doctors recorded that 'He supplied patients with a medicine superior to all their drugs, bottles and powders. That medicine was kindness and cheerful attention.' His poem *Come Up from the Fields, Father* is one of the greatest works of compassionate literature the War inspired.[5]

After Dickens and Whitman, there were several authors who qualified as doctors, and incorporated medicine into the background of much of their writing. Anton Chekhov said 'medicine is my lawful wife, and literature my mistress'. His father was the son of a serf and ran a grocery store. Chekhov had compassion. He made little money out of medicine, and treated the poor for free. Sadly, he died aged 44 from tuberculosis. Axel Munthe, the Swedish doctor who wrote *The Story of San Michelle* in 1929, was also a man of feeling. The book is a series of memoirs about many aspects of his life. Several chapters exude compassion. Munthe cared for the poor in the slums of Italy and Paris, and would not take money. He never wrote bills. Fortunately, he also had many wealthy patients, and the royalties from his books kept him in comfort. His description of the victims of the plague in Naples, and the earthquake in Sicily in 1908, are extremely moving. His concern for the dying is still palpable today.

About the same time in Britain there were three medical authors: Conan Doyle, A J Cronin and Somerset Maugham. Doyle's popular detective, Sherlock Holmes, epitomized the diagnostician solving mysteries. But it was Maugham's emotional novel *Of Human Bondage*, that was one of the most successful in its day. It was made into a film on three occasions.

A J Cronin was fiercely compassionate. He is best known in recent times for the television adaptation of *Dr Finley's Casebook*. But it has been claimed that his novel *The Citadel* prompted the establishment of the National Health Service in

CHAPTER 14

Drugs

There is a Chinese proverb, 'The beginning of wisdom is to call things by their correct name.' The medical vocabulary can sometimes confuse people with its ambiguities. Take the word 'abortion'. In gynaecology, it refers to any kind of failed pregnancy, a miscarriage, accidental or therapeutic. On the other hand, in the public mind, it refers exclusively to the pro-choice, pro-life debate.

The word 'drug' also has shades of meaning. In medicine, it refers to medication prescribed to patients with various conditions. In common usage, however, it often alludes to narcotics, or drugs of addiction. In sport, it may denote performance-enhancing drugs. Elsewhere, it may apply to so-called recreational drugs. These nuances of meaning in some ways reflect the changing perception of medicine in society.

In peering into the future of health care, we need to clarify our definitions. Consider the use and misuse of drugs in these diverse interpretations.

Chapter summary

- Medication
- Performance enhancement
- Narcotics
- Accidental overdose
- Recreational drugs
- Exercise addiction
- Conclusion

Medication

The therapeutic age began with the discovery of quinine. It is derived from the bark of the cinchona tree. Its medicinal properties were discovered by the Quechua Indians in Peru in the 17th century. Quinine was used to treat malaria until the 1940s, when more effective compounds were discovered.

Acetylsalicylic acid, commonly known as aspirin, was discovered in the 18th century and is still used today. The forerunner of aspirin, an extract of willow bark, had been around for a very long time. The therapeutic quality of this bitter-tasting astringent was noted in ancient Sumerian texts. Hippocrates recognized its value in reducing fever and relieving pain, as did native North American Indians.

In 1763, an English chaplain, Edward Stone, published a letter in the *Philosophical Transactions of the Royal Society*, recording the value of the bark of White Willow for the treatment of ague. But it was not until the end of the 19th century that the French chemist Charles Frederic Gerhardt produced the compound for the first time. By 1899, Bayer had manufactured and patented the drug. Since then, aspirin has been prescribed by the ton for over a century. Its analgesic, antipyretic, anti-inflammatory and blood-thinning qualities have been well documented. Even today, additional properties continue to be found. Like any drug, aspirin can have unwanted side effects, such as gastric haemorrhage, tinnitus or the childhood encephalopathy known as Reye's syndrome. Nonetheless, aspirin deserves a unique place in the history of medicine. Its discovery marked the beginning of the therapeutic age. One of the first drugs to be discovered, it was also one of the first to by-pass the doctor and be obtained over the counter (OTC), marking the beginning of DIY (Do It Yourself) medicine.

Shortly after Stone's discovery of the value of willow bark, William Withering in 1785 noticed that an elderly woman who practised as a folk herbalist used a remedy for dropsy (heart failure). Withering was a chemist, botanist and physician, and recognized that the active ingredient came from Witch's Glove, the foxglove plant. He called it by its Latin name, digitalis. Its discovery and use in cardiology is considered a milestone in pharmacology.

'Witch's Glove'[1]

Poem by Dr Michael E Scott (reproduced with permission)

Doctors knew the foxglove, *Digitalis purpurea*
was poisonous to animals, especially sheep and cattle,
so claims by simple folk that it might be a panacea
for failing hearts had been dismissed as foolish tittle tattle

A few believed a little of what harms may give relief,
but only Dr Withering put foxglove to the test.
In seventeen eighty five he publicised his firm belief –
of all herbs tried the powdered leaf of 'Witch's Glove' was best.

Dropsicals with racing hearts and moist nocturnal wheeze
passed large amounts of fluid, and regained their former verve,
could walk increasing distances and sleep with blissful ease.

Though then, as now, some patients suffered *Dig.* toxicity,
it's still in use, so Doctor William Withering deserves,
his place of honour on the roll of medicine's history.

It was another 60 years before the next important step. This was the discovery of anaesthesia. Many of the advances in anaesthesia were equally serendipitous, and go back generations to the use of opium. In the 19th century, alcohol had been used to induce stupefaction in wounded soldiers during the Crimean War. But the credit for the first use of modern anaesthesia goes, not to a physician, but to a dentist, William T G Morton. He demonstrated the use of ether, in the now famous ether dome of the Massachusetts General Hospital, in Boston on 16 October 1846.

The other compound that deserves a special place in the therapeutic age is insulin. Insulin is not a drug, but a physiological hormone, essential in intermediary metabolism. Its discovery revolutionized the treatment of diabetes. In 1921, a Canadian, Frederick Banting, had an idea for an experiment. He wrote a memo to himself: *'Ligate pancreatic ducts of the dog. Keep dogs alive till acini degenerate leaving islets. Try to isolate internal secretion of these and relieve glycosurea.'*

Banting, supported by Professor J J R Macleod, set about the experiment in Toronto, but needed one assistant. Two medical students, Charles Best and Clark Noble, tossed a coin for the summer job. Best won. Banting and Best, along with a biochemist, James Collip, went on to isolate insulin from the islets of Langerhans in the pancreas. (The islets had previously been identified by another medical student, Paul Langerhans, in Berlin in 1869.) The discovery was instantly dramatic. The trio went round a ward of dying diabetic children injecting them with the new compound. By the time they reached the end of their round, 'the first few were awakening from their coma, to the joyous exclamations of their families'. Banting and Macleod received the Nobel Prize for the discovery. Both graciously agreed to share the award with Best and Collip. Fully aware of the historical significance of their discovery, they all sold the patent to the university for a token of one dollar!

Several footnotes deserve mention in this remarkable story: Nicolae Paulescu, a Romanian physiologist, actually beat Banting and Best to the discovery by a short head, but the significance of his work with dogs went unrecognized. The other unfortunate loser was the student Clark Noble, who lost the coin toss for the Nobel Prize, an ironic twist in the spelling of his name. A question that might also be asked is, how long would the discovery have taken without the animal experiments?

The therapeutic age had arrived. The discovery of penicillin, a few years later, ushered in the pharmacological revolution that is well documented elsewhere.

Performance enhancement

The use of drugs to improve athletic performance is a relatively recent phenomenon. The practice quickly became widespread,[2] especially when professionalism entered the sport, with its financial incentives. Inevitably, physicians have been involved in the controversy.

Studies of track events from the 1936 Olympics in Berlin, when Jesse Owens won the 100 metres, onwards showed a steady improvement in performance over the years. Suddenly in the 1980s, there was a dramatic improvement, a quantum jump, in the times recorded. Doping had arrived.

Many different compounds have been used. Anabolic steroids are the most common. Cortisone was one of the first steroids to be isolated. Like insulin, it is a normal physiological substance. It has been used in medicine in therapeutic doses for decades. For a time, it was prescribed for so many conditions that it was labelled 'the last rites of 20th century medicine.' Gradually, many side effects of the large doses were identified. These include osteoporosis, diabetes and a moon-like facial appearance.

The anabolic steroids are synthetic derivatives of cortisone. They increase body mass, especially of muscle, and improve appetite and bone growth. One might easily guess from a glance at the muscular build of some athletes that perhaps not all of their 'Mr Atlas' physique has been acquired in the gymnasium. Again, numerous side effects have been identified. Many long-term effects may yet be uncovered. Tampering with the hormonal milieu is not advisable, and an eventual increase in the incidence of breast and prostate malignancy would not be surprising. More immediate dangers have been identified. In 2009, the death of a 17-year-old youth taking anabolic steroids was reported in Essex, England. Two people were arrested.

Athletes use many other drugs to improve their ability. Much of this is a grey area. For instance, runners from Kenya excelled in the Mexico City Olympics because of the high altitude. Nairobi is also elevated at 4000 feet. At these altitudes, the body develops a physiological polycythaemia, an increase in red cells, enhancing oxygenation. This can now be induced artificially by self-transfusion or with drugs.

Other drugs have been used to reduce stress, boost confidence, relieve athletic pain, or lose weight before weigh-in. Masking drugs have also been used to prevent detection of doping. Policing drug abuse in sport is an ongoing battle.

Narcotics

The word 'narcotic' is another ambiguous term. Strictly speaking, it refers to drugs that produce numbness and drowsiness – not to be confused with hypnotics, which are sleeping tablets, or analgesics, which are pain relievers. In medicine, the opioids have all three characteristics. In general use, however, the word 'narcotic' usually refers to illegal drugs, especially drugs of addiction. The opiates are derived from the opium poppy. The opioids include the opiates and their synthetic derivatives.

The opioids morphine, heroin (diamorphine) and their derivatives have a central place in medicine, particularly in terminal care. Heroin is especially useful in extreme cases. It is widely used in hospices in the UK, but there is a reluctance to use it in the USA because of the danger of illegal use.

Tackling drug addiction is a global problem. Addicts will pay anything to relieve their craving. They will steal if necessary. The market is immense. A billion dollar industry has built up a network of illegal supply, all the way from the source to the addict. Authorities struggle to intervene in the chain of destruction. Medicine's role has been largely limited to treatment and prevention. The brain loves the opioids.

'It lights up the limbic system, with cascading effects through the ventral striatum, midbrain, amygdala, orbitofrontal cortex and prefrontal cortex, leaving pure pleasure in its wake' (Kruger). But the scientific enigma of addiction remains.

Cocaine is also a drug of addiction. Although not in the same category as heroin, it is prohibited in most countries. Cocaine is derived from the leaves of the coca plant, and is a stimulant of the central nervous system. Its purest form is the powder crack cocaine. Many users believe that it is relatively harmless to health, but reports in 2010 confirm that cocaine accounts for 3% of sudden deaths.

The illegal drugs begin to merge into the recreational drugs.[3] These include Ecstasy (methylenedioxymethamphetamine), which has been used in psychotherapy; and LSD (lysergic acid diethylamide), which is a psychedelic drug. Marijuana, a hallucinogen, is however the most widely used recreational drug. Cannabis is derived from the hemp plant. Controlling the use of 'grass' or 'pot' is almost impossible as it can be grown in your backyard or bedroom.

The third group of drugs that deserve attention are the tranquillizers or anxiolytics. These consist mainly of the benzodiazepines, including diazepam, lorazepam and oxazepam. They provide short-term relief of anxiety. Dependence is common, and large numbers of people rely on these drugs.

The fourth group of drugs is used to control psychoses and depressive illnesses. They range from the phenothiazines to the newer generation agents.

Accidental overdose

The term 'overdose' in medicine often refers to attempted suicide. But a new phenomenon has emerged: accidental overdose due to opioid addiction. The relatively free availability of painkillers has resulted in a move from dependence to addiction for many patients. Pain deserved better treatment, and pain clinics emerged. Cathy Barber, of the Harvard School of Public Health, says, 'It was a compassionate change. Patient-advocacy groups pushed hard for it.' A range of drugs were prescribed, from simple codeine to oxycodone. Jeffrey Kluger[4] writes that 'no tooth extraction was complete, without a 30 day prescription for Vicodin [hydrocodone and paracetamol]. No ambulatory surgery ended without a trip to the hospital pharmacy to pick up some "oxy".' And often these scripts were renewable. One woman said, 'The doctor at the pain clinic didn't even ask my name at first. He wrote me a prescription while he was on the phone.'

The outcome was inevitable. Visits to accident and emergency units for unintentional overdoses soared. In 1990, there were about 6000 deaths in America from accidental drug poisoning. Public awareness of the problem was minimal and confined to celebrities, who were 'different'. But today there are seven deaths a day in Florida from prescription drug overdoses. Nationally, it is an epidemic. It is second only to road accidents as the leading cause of accidental death in the USA. No reliable figures are available in the UK.

Kluger says 'Big Pharma must help. That means climbing down off the opioid gravy train and working harder to develop more non-addictive painkillers – even if it means fewer sales and lower profits.' But the responsibility begins with the doctors who write the prescriptions.

Recreational drugs

'Recreational' is not so much a misnomer as a euphemism. Many of the drugs discussed above are used in social settings. By far the most common social drugs, however, are alcohol and tobacco. It is interesting that the rate of recidivism for both alcohol and nicotine is said to be the same as for heroin.

The attitude to alcohol in the USA has been a curiosity to non-Americans. The era of prohibition and bootlegging is a colourful part of the American legend. But how things have changed. Today in many states, alcohol can be bought over the counter, even in many of the larger pharmaceutical drug stores.

As far back as 1972, President Nixon commissioned Governor Raymond Shafer of Pennsylvania to chair the Report of the National Commission on Marihuana and Drug Abuse. One of the conclusions of that honest report was that, yes drug abuse is a problem, but it doesn't compare to the problem of alcohol and tobacco. Shafer noted that alcoholism afflicts nine million Americans, and accounts for many arrests, homicides, highway fatalities and huge economic costs. It wasn't what Nixon wanted to hear. He trashed the report and refused to read it.

Coincidentally, in Britain in 2009, the story was repeated by Professor David Nutt, Chairman of the Advisory Council on the Misuse of Drugs. He said Ecstasy, LSD and cannabis are less dangerous than both alcohol and tobacco. Once again, the government did not want to hear. Nutt deplored the artificial separation of alcohol and tobacco from illegal drugs. He said, 'No one is suggesting that drugs are not harmful. The critical question is one of scale and degree.' Nutt was sacked in October 2009 by the Labour Home Secretary, Alan Johnson.

A related problem is substance abuse. Strictly speaking, this refers to abuse or dependence on any non-medical drug. In practice, however, it usually refers to abuse of inhalants such as gasoline, aerosols or glue. Inhalant users tend to be people who do not have access to alcohol or other drugs, such as teenagers and incarcerated or institutionalized people. An exception is anaesthesia. For anaesthesiologists, it can be an occupational hazard. Previously, 'gas doctors' often sniffed the inhalant before sedating the patient, to check that the equipment was operating satisfactorily.

In passing, it should be noted that food can act as a tranquillizer. The top slimmer of 2009 describes food addiction. Bridie Coulter from North Ireland weighed 24 st 7 lb. She lost 14 st and went from dress size 34 to size 10. She said, 'I'd been overweight for my entire life, and the reason was that I always ate too much and never, ever did any exercise. I used to be like a drug addict but my habit was food. While I was ashamed of getting so big, the only thing that made me feel better was eating more.' Bridie had problems walking and breathing, and often slept on the living room sofa, as she lacked the energy to climb stairs to bed. Cured of her addiction, she says, 'You can't keep me still today.'

Exercise addiction

As a footnote to the discussion, a study by Professor Robin Kanarek,[5] at Tufts University in Boston, found that excessive running can be as addictive as heroin.

She noted that extreme exercise leads to a reaction in the brain similar to drug addiction. Sudden withdrawal leads to symptoms of 'cold turkey', including trembling, chattering teeth and drooping eyelids.

It is recognized that exercise produces chemicals known as beta-endorphins and dopamine that can lead to a 'high' after exercise.[6] Kanarek has added withdrawal symptoms to the syndrome. Scientists have suggested that exercise therapies may lead to new treatments for drug addicts, and may help for those who use excessive exercise to lose weight, an obsessive disorder now recognized as anorexia athletica.

Conclusion

The use and abuse of drugs has to be set in a wider context beyond medicine. As David Nutt and others discovered, the subject cannot be isolated from the political, economic, psychological and cultural forces in society.

References

1. Scott ME. Witch's Glove. *Irish Medical Journal* 2009; **102**: 229.
2. Ferstle J. Evolution and politics of drug testing. In: *Anabolic Steroids in Sport and Exercise*, 2nd edition (edited by Charles Yesalis). Human Kinetics: Champaign, IL, 2000: 363–414.
3. Lister S. LSD and ecstasy 'less dangerous than alcohol'. *The Times*, 29 October 2009.
4. Kluger J. The new drug crisis: addiction by prescription. *Time*, 13 September 2010.
5. Kanarek R. *Behavioural Science*, August 2009.
6. Alleyne R. Exercise as addictive as heroin. *The Daily Telegraph*, 19 August 2009.

CHAPTER 15

Medicalizing discontent and disease mongering

Chapter summary

- A panacea for everything
- Ageing as a disease: selling sickness
- Cosmetic surgery
- Botox

George Bernard Shaw made a distinction between normal eyesight and average eyesight. He noted that on average, older people develop presbyopia. This is not normal vision, in the sense that they need reading glasses. But it is a normal consequence of ageing. The concept has become warped, and has led to an insidious development in the pharmaceutical industry in recent years. It has been called the medicalization of discontent. Meika Loe, a sociologist in New York State, quotes sildenafil (Viagra) as a classic example.[1] Whereas reduced sex drive is common in older men, it has been redefined as abnormal. To create a market for Viagra, impotence was re-invented as erectile dysfunction. Men have been told they have a problem. A disease has been created. Healthy people are being bombarded by publicity telling them they are sick. Loe cites fluoxetine (Prozac) and methylphenidate (Ritalin) as other examples.

The ageing process is thus shorn of its physiological elements, creating a pathological condition that can be cured by medication. The problem is designed to fit the treatment, not the reverse.

The discovery of sildenafil is a classic case of serendipity. In a clinical drug trial for angina, it was discovered that an inevitable side effect was increased circulation to the genitalia. Pfizer suddenly had a product on their hands that deserved to be marketed. Loe says a sanitized medical campaign had to be created. Phallic malfunction was a possible euphemism. Then the advertising became more blatant. *'Get back to mischief'* was a caption on the Viagra website. Before long, vulgar Viagra jokes were everywhere: *'Viagra Extra Strength' – it even works at home.* The gags are easy to parody. One I have just conjured up: *'Viagra Lite' – recommended for stallions.*

With the longer lifespan in the population, there was a ready market for the drug. Hoping to exploit this even further, the pharmaceutical industry turned its attention to younger men. The demographic changed. In the USA, the marketing campaigns likened sexual performance to athletic ability. Viagra advertisements began to appear at baseball games.

Loe has applied George Ritzer's term, the 'McDonaldization' of America, to sex. She notes that the fast food ethic has pervaded our culture. Sex should be readily available, cheap, hot, and served up without delay. America's 'quick fix' pill culture provided a ready market. Again, the passage of legislation permitting direct-to-consumer advertising on television and on-line drug sales persuaded the public that there was a wider problem, cynically ensuring the expansion of the market, and profit from drug sales. Inevitably, rival drugs appeared on the market, with slightly different biochemical configurations to avoid using the same generic label. Vardenafil, co-marketed by Bayer, GlaxoSmithKline and Schering-Plough, was given the appropriate trade name of Levitra.

With the emancipation of women, the search is now on for a blockbuster drug for females. This is proving much more complex. Meanwhile, there is one statistic that is not advertised: 50% of men who have taken some of these drugs allegedly do not refill their prescriptions.

A panacea for everything

The concept has taken off and given rise to a whole new branch of pseudo-medicine, namely the medicalization of behavioural conditions.[2] The pharmaceutical industry is one of the largest and most profitable in the world. Marcia Angell writes, 'The drug companies have perfected a new and highly effective method to expand their markets. Instead of promoting drugs to fit diseases, they have begun to promote diseases to fit the drugs.' Instead of a pill for every ill, it is an ill for every pill. Some say we live in the pharmaceutical era.[3] The industry has considerable influence in the medical sphere, ranging from research and education to advertising and finance. People are increasingly turning to pills to solve their everyday anxieties and problems. Moreover, many doctors and health personnel are attached to pharmaceutical companies, either full time or in a part-time advisory capacity. And although doctors must declare conflicts of interest when publishing in recognized medical journals, there is no compulsion to do so in the sales world. The line between marketing and science has thus become blurred.

The list of behavioural conditions that has been explored for potential drug therapy is large. Alcoholism has been treated with a variety of medications for decades, with varying results. Today, drug therapy has been investigated for uses ranging from treatment of phobias to anger management. Some applications deserve careful consideration. For instance, a new drug has been discovered to prevent jet lag. Tasimelteon is said to shift the ebb and flow of the sleep hormone melatonin, thereby resetting the body's natural sleep rhythms. Not everyone who flies across a time zone needs medication, but no doubt its efficacy will be widely promoted.

Drugs have been devised for a number of more questionable conditions. They include the following 'disorders'.

Gambling

Topiramate, which is normally prescribed for epilepsy, has been used in one small study of 15 compulsive gamblers. It is claimed that over half found that the urge to gamble was controlled. In another study among gamblers, researchers at Yale University have investigated memantine, a drug used to treat the symptoms of Alzheimer's disease. It is thought that both of these drugs block the 'high' or buzz that comes with gambling.

Public speaking

Many people are extremely nervous when they have to speak in public. Some famous actors actually claim that this improves their performance. Lay speakers, however, sometimes feel paralysed and tongue-tied. Beta-blockers have been widely used in severe cases. The University of Minnesota has been testing the value of an antipsychotic drug known as quetiapine.

Anger management

Extreme cases of bad temper such as road rage or domestic violence have been labelled 'intermittent explosive disorder' (IED). It has been claimed that almost 10% of adults suffer from IED. Divalproex sodium (known outside the USA as valproate semisodium), a drug used for bipolar disorder and for seizure disorders, has been under investigation at the Mayo Clinic. Fluoxetine has also been used to treat aggression and induce calming.

Bereavement

Many physicians have been using antidepressants to treat those who have recently been bereaved. Currently, an investigation is underway to test the value of duloxetine in patients who have been devastated by the sudden unexpected death of a loved one.

Internet addiction

There is a fine line between spending time surfing the Internet and living on the Internet round the clock. Apparently, many do so at the cost of losing their social life, their jobs and even their wives! The antidepressant escitalopram has been used to treat cases at Mount Sinai Medical School in New York. Identical results were obtained with a placebo, however. A more serious problem, which can end up sending addicts to jail, is Internet pornography, especially if it involves children. Naltrexone has been tested at the Mayo Clinic.

Frigidity and dyspareunia

GlaxoSmithKline has been investigating bupropion to treat a condition known as inhibited female orgasm, thought to occur in one-third of women during their lifetime. As noted earlier, a drug for this problem could be another blockbuster like Viagra. At the same time, studies are ongoing to find a medication that would treat 'hypoactive sexual desire disorder'. Boehringer Ingelheim have studied flibanserin, a mood-altering compound. Sounds like an old fashioned aphrodisiac.

Phobias

Psycho-neurotic conditions range from anxiety states to obsessive–compulsive disorders, to claustrophobia and fears of many kinds. Most of these conditions have been treated with drugs for years, with varying results. Research continues, testing a number of compounds, and it is predicted that this field will expand considerably. Blushing and shyness have received special attention.

Shyness

Christopher Lane has written a book entitled *Shyness: How Normal Behavior Became a Sickness*.[4] He refers to the rapid increase in the number of psychiatric diagnoses, and the use of psychoactive drugs. As there are no objective tests for mental illness, and the boundaries between normal and abnormal are often hazy, he notes psychiatry is a particularly fertile field for creating new diagnoses and broadening old ones. Lane uses shyness as his case study of disease mongering. Shyness, as a psychiatric condition, first appeared in the textbooks as social phobia in 1980, but was rare. By 1994, it had become *social anxiety disorder*, now extremely common. According to Lane, one company decided to promote its antidepressant drug as treatment for social anxiety disorder, a severe medical condition. The slogan was *'Imagine being allergic to people.'* Sales soared. The product director was quoted as saying, 'Every marketer's dream is to find an unidentified or unknown market and develop it. That's what we were able to do with social anxiety disorder.'

Shoplifting

Perhaps the most bizarre 'condition' investigated for possible drug therapy is shoplifting. One of the most prominent 'patients' was the late Lady Isobel Barnett, a television personality on *What's My Line*. Isobel Barnett attended the prestigious Mount School in York, qualified in medicine, became a Justice of the Peace and married Sir Geoffrey Barnett. In 1980, she was found guilty of stealing a can of tuna and a carton of cream worth 87 pence. A few days later, she was found dead in her bath, having apparently committed suicide. This tragic situation is all too common. At the time of writing, four policemen have been accused of shoplifting: one in Sunderland, England, who quit the force, a second in Sweden, and a third on an American campus. A fourth, Detective Chief Inspector Jim Torbet, was arrested for shoplifting a bottle of wine. As with Isobel Barnett, he too committed suicide a few days later. The arguments will continue as to whether this incongruous behaviour is a crime, or a disease amenable to treatment with a new compound.

Memory pills

Medicines that were originally developed for Alzheimer's disease may soon be adapted for general use. Memory-enhancing pills are proving popular with some students to improve performance in examinations. These compounds have been called 'cognitive enhancing' or 'smart' drugs.[5]

Modafinil (Provigil) is a stimulant that has been used to treat narcolepsy, a condition in which patients keep falling asleep unexpectedly. Another stimulant, methylphenidate (Ritalin), which has been used to treat attention deficit disorder, has also been popular, amid claims that it promotes concentration. Adderall (a mixture of amphetamines) has also been favoured by many students. Undoubtedly, side effects will be observed with many of the newer drugs. Bouts of obsession have been reported in one case. A worry is that it is possible to obtain these drugs from the Internet without prescription, before they have been fully tested.

Memory-blocking pills

And if it is unhappy or embarrassing memories that you wish to erase, a pill may be on the way.[6] Workers in Switzerland have developed a drug that dissolves the sheath around the amygdala in the brain of animals, an area where fearful memories are stored. Human brains have similar sheaths, and such a drug might help people wipe out fearful memories, overwriting them with happy thoughts. Moralists have been concerned that confession may be a thing of the past.

Warfare: shell shock and PTSD

Arguably the most controversial use of mood-altering drugs is in warfare, especially by the US armed forces. The folly of the First World War has been debated over the years. At the time, a German general famously said of the British troops that they were 'lions led by donkeys'. Hundreds of soldiers were shot at dawn for desertion and cowardice (see box). Ben McIntyre of *The Times* said 'Many of those who were executed in The Great War did not receive justice, even by the standards of the day.' One was shot for overstaying his seven-day marriage leave. At least four were under-age *volunteers*. In some cases, soldiers in the firing squad who refused to shoot were themselves shot at dawn as an example. It was only after years of agitating that the Shot at Dawn Campaign succeeded in persuading the British government to change its stance. In November 2006, it was agreed that all soldiers executed for military offences should be given a conditional pardon.

MILITARY EXECUTIONS
Shot at dawn, First World War

France	600
Italy	500
Britain	346
Germany	48
Canada	25
Belgium	13
USA	10
New Zealand	5
Australia	Nil
Russia	Nil

Shell shock or battle fatigue has now been redefined as combat stress reaction, or post-traumatic stress disorder (PTSD). Having been given a psychiatric diagnostic label, it was a green light for drug therapy. Before long, the Pentagon quietly agreed to the use of antidepressants in combat troops. Between 10% and 20% of the American armed forces in Iraq and Afghanistan were on prescription medications.

Historically, the use of drugs to bolster the troops is not a new idea. Officers ordered rum rations for Union troops in the American Civil War. More recently the Luftwaffe used amphetamines in the Second World War.

Medication is alleged to alleviate the intolerable distress suffered by military personnel caught up in the horror of warfare. *Time* magazine quotes a military doctor who said, 'Boy it's really nice to have these drugs, so that we can keep people redeployed.' But one soldier who was on medication in Baghdad said that PTSD isn't fixed by taking medication. It is just numbed. He added that he felt drugged all the time. One study by the Rand Corporation suggests that at best the effects are modest.

This sounds familiar. The results of most drug trials are at best modest. The role of medicine to help soldiers slaughter the enemy is a new departure for the profession. But the pharmaceutical companies are not going to argue.

Interestingly, drugs may not be the best way of dealing with anxiety in the armed forces. For some years, 'lack of moral fibre' was known by the initials LMF, and was a charge against airmen in the Second World War. Many personnel with the condition had to be discharged from service. However, after counselling and support in the RAF, two-thirds of those afflicted were able to return to flying. This compared with zero who had no support in the US Army Air Force.

Living

As already noted, the influence of the pharmaceutical industry is pervasive. No longer is it 'a pill for every ill', but rather 'an ill for every pill'. And more: why not a pill for living itself?

When it was discovered that tamoxifen had a beneficial effect on patients with estrogen-receptor (ER)-positive breast cancer, it was proposed that perhaps it should be given to healthy women who might be at risk some time in the future. Again, when it was found that statins helped lower cholesterol in those with abnormal raised levels, it was soon suggested that rosuvastatin (Crestor) also be given to those with normal or even low cholesterol. The surprise was that this paper was given credence in the *New England Journal of Medicine*, even though the principal author openly admitted that he was in association with the pharmaceutical company.

The idea has also grown that Prozac *can make you feel better than well*. The pursuit of happiness is an elusive goal. Philosophers, psychologists and gurus might argue that happiness is a by-product, not an end in itself. But why not a happiness pill? Aldous Huxley explored his experiences with mescaline and LSD in *Brave New World*. Opium has been used for generations, especially in the East, alcohol for even longer everywhere. All have side effects, often unpleasant, sometimes fatal. In an age where celebrities are revered more than Nobel laureates, and celebrity magazines sell millions of copies per issue, it is hardly surprising that the celebrity culture prospers. One can only hope that the spirit of man will survive the onslaught – but the prospect is not bright.

Ageing as a disease: selling sickness

The story of how 'osteopenia' was categorized as a disease has been told by Alix Spiegel on National Public Radio (NPR) in the USA.[7] It illustrates the marketing phenomenon in health care.

Katie Benghauser, a fit 54-year-old American woman, went to her doctor for a check-up. She was a model of health and could outrun most 20-year-olds. Yet because her sister had some bone problems, and because Katie herself was a female of slight frame, she might be at future risk of osteoporosis. A bone density test was ordered. Back came the result: osteopenia.

When clinicians see the word osteopenia, they think that it's a disease. What should they do? The answer must be medication. Actually, osteopenia is a slight thinning of the bones, which occurs naturally as women get older, and typically does not lead to bone fractures.

Twenty years ago, the diagnosis of osteoporosis was 'all over the map'. Experts could not decide where to draw the line on a graph of bone density. Apparently, more or less off the cuff, at an international conference in a hotel room in Rome, a line was drawn, and every woman on one side had the disease. The question was, how do you describe women on the other side of the line? Someone coined the term osteopenia.

Alendronic acid (Fosamax) was the first non-hormonal drug that was found to slow the progression of osteoporosis. Why not prescribe it for osteopenia? The story of how this came about and how the drug was marketed is compelling. First, osteopenia had to be diagnosed. Bone density machines that measured the spine and hip were too expensive for most doctors' offices in the USA. But peripheral machines were small and portable and could measure the wrist, forearm and heel. Eventually Medicare in the USA was persuaded to reimburse bone scan measurements. From there on, it was all downhill. Bone densitometry became increasingly available. Steve Cummings, a Director of Clinical Research in California, said that it became 'almost viral'. Everyone wanted the test. Screening examinations soared from 77,000 in 1994 to 1.5 million in five years.

Two men involved in the debate on bone density problems disagree. Richard Mazess, of the Lunar Corporation, argues that many were 'compliant in a plot to misdiagnose American women'. On the other hand, Jeremy Allen, involved in promoting the work, believes that he helped save millions of lives.

NPR says that the paradox of the health care system is that both these men are probably right. Drug companies produce drugs that relieve suffering, but, in order to profit from them, they need to extend their use to as many people as possible. That frequently means to milder and milder forms of the disease.

There is a powerful economic incentive to expand the boundaries between health and disease. This is evident in many areas, from the cholesterol saga, to the margin between sadness and depression. Many branches of medicine merge imperceptibly from the physiological to the pathological. In the end, ageing itself has been diagnosed as a disease.

Cosmetic surgery

It is not only physicians who have been caught up in this maelstrom. Take the wholly admirable specialty of plastic surgery, now entangled with the cosmetic industry, surgerizing ageing itself. It is no longer acceptable to grow old gracefully. W B Yeats wrote presciently 'No country for old men', a phrase that was picked up by Cormac McCarthy in his novel and later in an Oscar-winning film. Yeats could have added, nor old women.

Plastic surgeons became well known in wartime when they perfected skin grafting for patients disfigured with burns and horrific injuries. As the specialty progressed, the work expanded to develop various prosthetic procedures. In my own field, breast reconstruction is now offered routinely to many patients following lumpectomy or mastectomy for breast cancer. Not all women are keen to undergo the procedure, however. One prominent nursing writer wrote in the *Lancet*, 'Women of my age are more concerned with concealing their bottoms, than revealing their tops.'

In 2008, at their Annual Conference, The British Association of Aesthetic Plastic Surgeons (BAAPS) deplored the misleading advertising and marketing practices of certain clinics.[8] These included lunchtime facelifts and the use of models with anatomically impossible breasts. One even offered a £250 discount to customers as an incentive to have prompt surgery. Some years ago, such blatant advertising would have led to surgeons being struck off the register. The General Medical Council (GMC) no longer has control over this, and the BAAPS is not a regulatory body. Only one-third of plastic surgeons are members of the BAAPS. The general Advertising Standards Authority has some teeth, but so far seems more concerned about food products and soap powders.

A report in September 2010 by The National Confidential Enquiry into Patient Outcome and Death found fundamental weaknesses in the way cosmetic surgery is carried out in the UK.[9] Too many teams were prepared to 'have a go' at procedures they rarely performed. The two-stage process, which allows patients to reflect on treatment beforehand, was not performed in about two-thirds of cases. Half the operating theatres were not properly equipped, and there was no emergency back-up. Dr Alex Goodwin, the report author, said 'failure to monitor patients after surgery is a recipe for disaster'. Amanda Sherlock, Director of Operations in the new Care Quality Commission (CQC), said, 'It is unacceptable some centres don't have the basic standards of good medical practice.' And Peter Walsh, Chief Executive of Action against Medical Accidents, said 'shabby treatment is putting lives at risk'. The Department of Health added, 'The findings cast "a long shadow" over the industry', and they can expect tougher legislation. The new CQC will be able to fine and prosecute the worst offenders.

Interestingly, Americans could be facing a tax on cosmetic surgery, to help pay for the enormous costs of proposed changes in health care. Senators have proposed a 10% levy on breast implants, nip and tuck tummy surgery, facial lifts, hair transplants, and teeth whitening. Americans spent $7 billion on cosmetic procedures in 2008. Critics say such a tax would be discriminatory, since it would disproportionately affect women, who make up over 80% of cosmetic patients. But it may not happen. New Jersey previously introduced a similar law, but repealed it, since it only collected one-quarter of the expected revenue.

The concept of a tax on these procedures is intriguing. It implies that beauty enhancement is part of the cosmetic industry, not the treatment of disease.

Botox

Perhaps the most unusual branch of cosmetic medicine is the Botox industry. It is difficult for a man to write about it, although some men do undergo injections. Botulinum toxin type A is derived from the bacterium *Clostridium botulinum*. It is a highly toxic substance that is responsible for the illness botulism, which may be caused by ingestion of bacterially contaminated food or by contamination of wounds. Botox is the brand name for a medicinal form of the substance. It is a dilute purified very low-concentration form of the toxin.

When injected in tiny doses directly into muscles, the toxin blocks the chemical signals that cause muscles to contract. The skin then relaxes and becomes smoother. Botox is widely used to 'treat' facial wrinkles and 'crow's feet'.

Side effects are unusual, although rarely the compound can spread and cause serious systemic symptoms. Occasionally also, patients may end up with facial asymmetry and facial weakness. The main problem is that the effect is temporary and only lasts about six months. Injections then have to be repeated to maintain the results, and in that sense can become 'addictive'.

Botox injections have also been used for excessive sweating in hyperhydrosis, and more importantly, for relaxing muscles in cerebral palsy. Botox is now the most common cosmetic procedure in Britain and the USA. The average cost for a course of treatment varies between $350 and $500.

There is some concern that unqualified rogue practitioners may be offering the procedure. It is perhaps difficult to claim, however, that the technique calls for a lengthy medical education. A tattooist is hardly appropriate, but a specially trained dental surgeon, or highly qualified nurse practitioner, could presumably be trained to administer the injections.

Ageing is not a disease and growing old not a disorder. Perhaps the best that can be said for the merger between cosmetics and medicine comes from the Hippocratic corpus: *Primum nil nocere* – First do no harm.

References

1. Loe M. *The Rise of Viagra. How the Little Blue Pill Changed Sex in America*. New York University Press: New York, 2004.
2. Dobson R. Behavioural issues. A cure for everything. *Belfast Telegraph*, 5 June 2008.
3. Pearson M. *Our Daily Meds. How the Pharmaceutical Companies Transformed Themselves into Slick Marketing Machines and Hooked the Nation on Prescription Drugs*. Sarah Crichton Books/Farrar, Straus and Giroux: New York, 2008.
4. Lane C. *Shyness: How Normal Behavior Became a Sickness*. Yale University Press, 2008.

5. Cockcroft L. 'Memory pill' that could help with exam revision could be available soon. *The Daily Telegraph*, 18 January 2009.
6. Harlow J. Drug may wipe out troubling memories. *The Sunday Times*, 13 September 2009.
7. Spiegel A. How a bone disease grew to fit the prescription. *National Public Radio (NPR)*, 21 December 2009.
8. Cosmetic surgery ad clampdown. *BBC News*, 19 September 2008.
9. Triggle N. Cosmetic surgery industry in UK 'has key weaknesses'. *BBC News Health*, 16 September 2010.

CHAPTER 16

Pharmaceutical profits: trials and tribulations

I t is recognized that doctors can no longer police themselves. The same is true of the pharmaceutical industry. The pharmaceutical lobby, also known as Big Pharma, has a fundamental dilemma: the conflict between basic science and commercial interest. Altruism

Chapter summary

- KOLs
- Unwanted side effects

is a noble goal, but to survive in the business world you have to make a profit. The success of the pharmaceutical industry in advancing health care is one of the great triumphs of our time. Unfortunately, there has also been a downside, involving a number of clinical disasters that have led to calls for greater regulation than at present exists.

The thalidomide catastrophe made headlines in 1961. Again in 2006, the side effects observed in young volunteers in the Northwick Park 'Elephant Man' clinical trial in London were disastrous. All six participants, testing a drug for rheumatoid arthritis, were admitted to intensive care with suspected organ failure. Two were in a serious condition. One of the victims' head ballooned in size, and he had several toes amputated. His sobbing girlfriend said he resembled the elephant man. One expert said the men might never fully recover.

Several other problems with clinical trials have emerged more recently. In one case, a prominent drug company in the USA set up a phase I drug trial. It transpired that the so-called healthy volunteers were neither healthy nor volunteers.[1] They were in fact homeless alcoholics. In another case in Europe, one volunteer eager to earn a little extra entered two separate trials at the same time.

In India, 49 babies died in a trial used to test experimental drugs.[2] India has become the leading destination for international pharmaceutical companies to outsource clinical trials. Manish Tiwari, a spokesperson for the Congress Party in India in 2008, was incensed and said, 'the practice of using infants like guinea-pigs for drug testing must end.'

Part of the problem is the pressure to bring new drugs onto the market. The frequent reports of 'breakthroughs' in the media, not only in the tabloids but also the broadsheets, have prompted an emotional campaign for providing expensive drugs of marginal benefit for every dying patient. The previous question was: what is the cost of a human life? The more precise question now is: what is the cost of extending life by a few more months? The answer is: a lot.

The case of Abigail Burroughs is pertinent. This 21-year-old American woman died of squamous carcinoma of the head and neck in 2001. This is a hideous condition and a distressing way to die. Abigail's anguished father claimed that she died prematurely. He said there were drugs available that might have helped. These drugs were in experimental phase I clinical trials. He founded the Abigail Alliance for better access to experimental drugs. The Washington DC circuit court ruled that a patient with terminal illness had a fundamental right under the constitution to experimental drugs in phase I trials. The case had wide-reaching implications. It is often difficult to be certain of the benefit of a drug in the early stages of a phase III trial, never mind phase I. The case was rejected on appeal, for it would have opened the door to chaotic demands for unproven medications.

More disturbing was the report in 2008 that Dr Joseph Biederman, a prominent child psychiatrist at Harvard, received $1.6 million from drug companies.[3] Dr Biederman spearheaded a massive increase in the diagnosis of bipolar disorders in children.[4] These children, some as young as two years old, were being treated with a cocktail of powerful drugs. Biederman's considerable international reputation promoted these mind-altering medications, resulting in vast revenues for drug companies. Failing to disclose this conflict of interest prompted an investigation by Senator Charles Grassley on the Senate Finance Committee. Two of Dr Biederman's colleagues, Dr Timothy Wilens and Dr Thomas Spencer, belatedly reported earning at least $1 million after being pressed by Senator Grassley.

More recently, it was discovered that prominent physicians in other centres were also receiving huge sums from pharmaceutical companies,[5] and there is now widespread concern about conflicts of interest in many cases. The Chicago psychiatrist Dr Michael Reinstein has been at the centre of a debate about the efficacy and side effects of Seroquel (quetiapine), an antipsychotic drug manufactured by AstraZeneca. Reinstein was a leading figure in conducting research into Seroquel that made its results look spectacular.[6] AstraZeneca paid him almost half a million dollars over a decade to travel the nation promoting the drug.[7]

In Britain, Dr John Blenkinsopp, AstraZeneca's former UK medical manager, claimed that he was pressurized by the company's marketing arm to approve claims about the drug that he felt did not reflect the medical evidence.[8]

Blowing the whistle on pharmaceutical companies is fraught with difficulty. A report in the *New England Journal of Medicine* in 2010 notes that Pfizer paid $2.3 billion in the USA to settle allegations that it marketed its drugs illegally to physicians, leading to unnecessary payments by the government.[9] The authors interviewed 26 whistle blowers involved in drug company cases between 2001 and 2009. Twenty-two were insiders referred to as realtors. Whistle blowers are sometimes portrayed as heroes struggling against corporate greed, but others question their motives and the 'excessive' rewards that they sometimes receive. Most tried to resolve the problems internally, and only went public reluctantly when all else failed. Although many made large sums of money, the majority concluded that the personal cost to their lives and careers was not worth the struggle

Dr Fiona Godlee, Editor of the *BMJ*, says that sometimes submissions for drug approval 'are buried in truckloads of information'. At present in Britain, the regulator – the Medicines and Health Care Products Regulatory Authority (MHRA) – has to rely on research provided by the drug companies when it licenses a medicine. Godlee says the only solution is to have new drugs tested by an independent body. She adds that even the most avid Manchester United supporter would not have Alex Ferguson refereeing a match. But the MHRA maintains that it carries out detailed reviews of all applications. So the arguments continue.

KOLs

Influential doctors are referred to by the industry as 'thought leaders' or 'key opinion leaders' ('KOLs'). They are of immense value to the pharmaceutical industry, and not surprisingly are handsomely rewarded. In return, the industry has extensive ties to physicians, and to senior faculty members, in prestigious medical schools.

In a review of three books on the influence of drug companies in clinical trials, Dr Marcia Angell (former editor of the *New England Journal of Medicine*) says that companies often insist, as a condition of funding, that they must be involved in the research programme. Thus, bias can easily be introduced in trials, to make products look better than they are. For instance, a drug that is likely to be used in the elderly may be tested in younger patients, so that side effects are less likely to emerge. Angell notes that medical investigators are often little more than hired hands, collecting data according to the requirements of the company.

Alison Bass has shown how favourable results are sometimes published, and unfavourable results buried.[10] It has also been noted that when the results of trials are submitted to the Food and Drug Administration (FDA) in America, if one or two trials are positive – that is, show efficacy without serious risk – the drug is approved, even if all other trials are negative.[11]

A separate report in Europe, published in the *Annals of Oncology*, stated that exaggerated claims are being made for new cancer treatments that are not justified by the evidence.[12] A number of trials were halted prematurely to deliver rapid results. A total of 25 trials were stopped early, because they started to show benefit before statistical significance had been obtained. The authors, at the Mario Negri Institute for Pharmacological Research in Milan, said, 'This suggests a commercial component in marketing these drugs.' Some of the most well-known chemotherapy agents were cited in the report, including trastuzumab (Herceptin), irinotecan (Campto) and bevacizumab (Avastin).

Commenting on the article, the Editor of the *Annals of Oncology*, Professor David Kerr, said, 'Researchers face a dilemma. If we see an effective drug, it is our duty to get it into the clinic as quickly as possible. But we must not run down the quality of the evidence to support that drug.' The *Lancet* went further in 2004 and accused pharmaceutical companies of 'confusion, manipulation and institutional failure'. A kinder interpretation is to call it 'wish bias'.

In the USA, drugs are only approved for a specific purpose, and it is illegal for companies to promote them for anything else. But it is possible for doctors to prescribe approved drugs, 'off label', that is, without regard to their specified use, and this is frequently done.

Moreover, it has been noted that even universities and institutes may have a conflict of interest, where physicians bring in massive funding, including endowment of chairs. As a result, such bodies are hardly in a position to object to faculty members behaving in the same way. Thus, oversight is lax and permissive, and the rules are only loosely enforced.

In the case of Dr Biederman, the president of the Massachusetts General Hospital, and the chairman of its physician organization, sent a letter to the physicians involved, expressing, not shock over the enormity of conflict of interest, but sympathy for the beneficiaries:[3] *'We know this is an incredibly painful time for these doctors and their families, and our hearts go out to them.'*

But it is not only the big names who promote the new products. When the custom of drug companies giving gifts to doctors was banned, a new commercial ruse was devised. A doctor with a large practice is invited to become an educator. He is given a set of slides and coached on the merits of the latest medication. He is then paid a modest sum of say $1,500 to lecture a roomful of doctors over dinner and wine.

The doctor may believe that he has been recruited to persuade his colleagues to consider the merits of the new drug.[13] He doesn't realize that he himself is the primary target. Afterwards, his prescribing habits are tracked. Often, he unwittingly writes a series of prescriptions for the expensive new product. One whistleblower said we would see a speaking doctor write an additional $100,000 to $200,000 in prescriptions. As one rep remarked, 'It's a good return on the investment.' It is almost impossible for a reputable physician to recognize that he has been influenced – some might say manipulated.

Unwanted side effects

There are very few drugs that are completely free of unwanted side effects. Even aspirin, which has been prescribed by the ton for over a century, can cause catastrophic gastric haemorrhage in adults, or Reye's syndrome in children. Cytotoxic cancer drugs are one degree worse. They are cell poisons by definition. Nonetheless, advances in pharmacology have improved the lives of millions, albeit at some cost to others.

One of the most profitable areas in the pharmaceutical industry is the development of anticancer drugs, particularly the monoclonal antibodies. Yet some of the claims may have been exaggerated. Currently for instance, it is suggested that cancer could be transformed in the next 20 years from a fatal condition to a manageable one like diabetes. The comparison is flawed, however. Diabetes is controlled by injecting a normal physiological compound, insulin. Cancer is a disease of cellular anarchy. Although progress has been rapid and the outlook is favourable, there is no evidence, so far, that it is simply a matter of replacing a single missing compound.

At the same time, pharmaceutical companies have to promote their products in a highly competitive market place. The success rate in the development of cancer drugs improved in 2009 from a previous 5% to 18%. This improvement has been largely due to the switch in research strategy from rational empiricism to molecular targeting, with the development of designer drugs. But there is still a huge failure rate of over 80%. Many promising compounds have to be abandoned for a variety of reasons, including drug instability and unacceptable side effects. Inevitably, this increases the costs of new drugs, and these have to be recouped.

The conflict between commercial interests and ethics persists. Clearly, patient welfare must come first. Sadly, however, a degree of cynicism is emerging. One pharmaceutical marketing executive allegedly said that their job is to convince Americans that there are only two kinds of people: *'Those with medical conditions that require drug treatment, and those who don't know it yet.'*

Marcia Angell states that 'If the medical profession does not put an end to this form of corruption voluntarily, it will lose the confidence of the public, and the government will step in and impose legislation.' Another nail in the coffin of the profession.

References

1. Elliott C. Guinea-pigging. Should people take drugs for a living? Department of Medical Ethics. *The New Yorker*, 7 January 2008
2. Blakely R. Drug trials under investigation after 49 babies die at leading hospital. *The Times*, 20 August 2008.
3. Angell M. Drug companies and doctors: a story of corruption. *The New York Review of Books*, 15 January 2009.
4. Harris G, Carey B. Researchers fail to reveal full drug pay. *The New York Times*, 8 June 2008.
5. Harris G. Leading psychiatrists didn't reveal full drug pay. *The New York Times*, 4 October 2008.
6. Jewitt C. Pro Publica and Pharma Gossip. New York, 11 November 2009.
7. Roe S. The Seroquel scandal. *The Chicago Tribune*, 27 October 2009.
8. Alexander A. Whistleblower claims drug test data suppressed. *BBC File on Four*, 26 January 2010.
9. Kesselheim A, Studdert D, Mello M. Whistleblowers' experiences in fraud litigation against pharmaceutical companies. *New England Journal of Medicine* 2010; **362**: 1832–9.
10. Bass A. *Side Effects: A Prosecutor, a Whistleblower, and a Bestselling Antidepressant on Trial.* Algonquin Books of Chapel Hill: Chapel Hill, NC, 2008.
11. Negative drug research withheld. *BBC News*, 23 April 2004.
12. Trotta F, Apolone G, Garattini S, Tafuri G. Stopping a trial early in oncology: for patients or for industry? *Annals of Oncology* 2008; **19**: 1347–53.
13. Spiegel A. How to win doctors and influence prescriptions. *National Public Radio (NPR)*, 21 October 2010.

CHAPTER 17

Nursing grievances

The importance of traditional nursing

The evolution of the nursing profession has been one of the big advances in health care. It has merged imperceptibly into medicine in many areas, in general practice, midwifery and obstetrics, anaesthesia, and screening for disease. But there has been a downside.

Many deplore the loss of traditional nursing care, listening to the patient, the cheerful disposition, holding the hand of the sick and infirm – yes, and making the bed and washing the patient.

The move towards the administrative nurse with a university degree began in America and moved to Britain and Ireland. It has now been proposed that all British nurses should enrol in a degree course. This is a mistake, if it excludes those who want to pursue a vocation, rather than an academic qualification. One criticism is that the graduate nurse has been busy meeting administrative targets, and filling out forms, instead of attending to patients' everyday needs. We have to be careful not to leave traditional nursing behind.

In 2009, the Patients Association in the UK published a report detailing the decline in nursing care. It made shocking reading. It revealed that patients were often left in soiled bedclothes, and those unable to feed themselves were left without food, and even abused in some cases. Some aspects of the report were appalling. Old people were neglected, lying in their own faeces, hungry and afraid, while nurses chatted callously at the nursing station, indifferent to the suffering of those around them.

It also transpired that many of the traditional roles were left to health care assistants and nursing auxiliaries. In some instances, these assistants had as little as one week of training. Worse, many were employed in high-dependency units, charged with checking blood sugar levels, measuring blood pressure and recording electrocardiographs. Moreover, they were often dressed in uniforms that made it difficult to distinguish them from qualified nurses. It has been alleged that this little deception might even be deliberate, to confuse patients and relatives about staffing levels. The background to this is an administrative dodge to save cash on the wards.

At the same time, criticism has been made of ambitious nurses who perceive more menial tasks to be beneath them.[1] One nurse reportedly told another, 'Washing is not part of your job. It is not part of your job description.' In another instance, in a letter to the London *Daily Telegraph*, Madeleine Burton, a nurse, wrote how a fellow student in her former nursing class declared, 'I did not train for three years to feed and bathe someone.' Burton added that this nurse was chosen as 'student of the year'!

Claire Rayner, President of the Patients Association, and a former nurse and newspaper agony aunt, admitted that such views were widely held by nurses. 'It is an appalling attitude to say it is not your job to wash patients. I am afraid this is spreading widely and I disapprove of it strongly. Unfortunately today's nurses think it is too menial.'

Minette Marrin, writing in the *Sunday Times*, is even more outspoken. She draws attention to 'the fallen angels', the nightmare or devil nurses, protected by silence. She says 'many are slovenly with loose hair hanging over patients' wounds, unkempt nails, and hands rarely washed between patients. And many are just mean.' What has happened?

In response, Glynis Pellatt, a lecturer in nursing, says that it is wrong to think that nurse training in the past was superior. She says that the old apprenticeship style exploited student nurses as cheap labour. Eighteen-year-old students were commonly left on the wards at night with one nursing auxiliary. She admits, however, that 'uncaring neglectful nurses are a disgrace'.

The problems with nursing are not confined to Britain. An acquaintance visiting the USA was admitted to hospital with a ruptured appendix. He was full of praise for the surgical team. However, his postoperative nursing care was appalling. One nurse's fingernails were so long that she was unable to put on the rubber gloves. He promptly signed himself out of hospital against advice, and returned to Europe in haste.

Sadly, the influx of uncaring nurses, only interested in earning a wage, ignores those dedicated nurses who devote their working lives to caring for the sick. To paraphrase a lyric,

> *Nurses, who used to do caring,*
> *Aren't nursing any more.*
> *They're doing bibliography.*

It was inevitable that nurses with a university qualification should move with the times. Not surprisingly, they began to spend more time at the nursing station, distancing themselves from the patients. The administrative load that qualified nursing staff have to deal with is unconscionable. It is partly due to the plague of litigation. Every last fart has to be recorded in the report. Somewhere, a balance has to be achieved. The nursing profession should be encouraged to develop a career structure. At present, there is a glass ceiling, and the only way up is to head into administration and bureaucracy. It is moving in the wrong direction.

Specialization in nursing care

The trend towards specialization with the nurse practitioner is a better road to take, towards medicine itself. Training should begin at the bedside, chatting up the patients, listening to their concerns, moving on to record the vital signs of temperature, pulse, blood pressure and level of consciousness, and performing technical investigations.

How far the role should be extended is a matter for debate. The terms 'nurse practitioner', 'nurse specialist' and even nurse consultant have emerged. Clare Lomas, writing in *Nursing Times* in 2009, notes that the boundaries between doctors and nurses have become blurred.[2] Pregnant women can self-refer themselves to midwives, bypassing the GP. The first nurse-led walk-in clinic in Britain opened in January 2000. Since then, some nurse specialists have been able to order *and interpret* diagnostic tests, prescribe medication, and discharge patients from hospital.[3]

The Calman Report in 1991 recommended that appropriately trained nurses could extend their roles to take on tasks previously carried out by doctors, in effect becoming substitute doctors, although this term is avoided. It was claimed that improving nurse practitioner skills 'promotes personal development, and encourages career enhancement'. The move inevitably involves additional study and training. Not everyone agrees that it is cost-effective.

Nonetheless, the changes are already well underway.[4] Nurse endoscopists now perform osephago-gastro-duodenoscopy (OGD), flexible sigmoidoscopy, colonoscopy and even biopsies. In a multi-institution study of endoscopies performed by nurses, 'no significant differences between doctors and nurses undertaking upper and lower GI endoscopies were found, except that patients were more satisfied with nurses after one day'. Again, Dr Jan Koornstra found nurse-performed colonoscopy to be effective and safe in a study of 100 cases in the Netherlands. Similar results have been found for nurses performing colposcopies in gynaecology.

Nurse-led follow-up cancer clinics have been pioneered in oncology. In a more ambitious move, the nurse practitioner role has been extended to undertake advanced intervention procedures, including a form of Nd:YAG (neodymium-doped yttrium aluminium garnet) laser peripheral iriditomy.

A degree of caution has been recommended. Anne-Marie Rafferty, Professor of Nursing Policy and Dean of King's College London's Florence Nightingale School of Nursing and Midwifery, says that there has to be a clear division of labour, and effective communication between nurses and doctors. Failure-to-care situations often occur where there is confusion about roles, and lack of communication. Dr Shree Datta of the British Medical Association agrees that there needs to be a distinction between the roles of doctors and nurses, to ensure that priorities are allocated correctly. She adds that the lines of communication have to remain open, or there is potential for conflict. The professional bodies have to be clear on the remit, to ensure complementary working and mutual respect.

Beyond that, it is always possible for nurses who wish to pursue further studies to enrol in medical school. There have been a number of precedents, most famously Dame/Nurse/Doctor Cicely Saunders.

Meanwhile, someone has to deal with the incontinent patient. Auxiliaries should not have a monopoly of these unpleasant tasks. Student nurses should start at the bottom, literally and metaphorically. And why exclude junior medical students from starting with these chores?

High-tech medicine has yet to devise a method of emptying the bedpan. If we can get to the Moon, why is it so difficult to devise such a device? There is money to be made by some entrepreneur.

Perhaps the time has come to recognize the changing nursing scene and distinguish between the different roles. We need both the carers and the curers. It is difficult to do both in a 24-hour day. A new name is needed to go with the academic/administrative nurse, not paramedic, not nurse specialist, not nurse consultant. There are precedents for the specialized nurse: the midwife in Europe, or the anaesthetist in America. The Russian title *feldsher* seems entirely appropriate for the new role.

Meanwhile, the vocational nurse should not be forgotten. Let us reserve the title of nurse for those who are involved in bedside nursing and caring for the sick. And we all know who that is when we are ill. Raymond Tallis, Emeritus Professor of Geriatric Medicine at Manchester University, says that his 'concern for the lonely frightened patient sitting in a pool of urine, is not entirely disinterested. One day it will be me. Or you.'[5]

As medical science continues its assault on premature disease, and life expectancy is extended, the role of the doctor may diminish, but the need for nursing care will increase. We are going to need more, many more, vocational nurses, not fewer. The emphasis is moving from medical care to nursing care, not the other way round.

References

1. Kate-Templeton S. Nurses are 'too clever' to care for you. *The Times*, 24 April 2004.
2. Doctors and nurses: blurring the boundaries. *Nursing Times*, 29 September 2009.
3. Stott F, Barnett S, Hester N. Nurses, degrees and the death of GP practices. Correspondence. *The Times*, 14 November 2009.
4. Williams J, Russell I, Durai D et al. Effectiveness of nurse delivered endoscopy: findings from randomised multi-institution endoscopy trial (MINuET). *BMJ* 2009; **338**: b231.
5. Tallis R. How will a degree help a frightened patient? *The Times*, 13 November 2009.

The demarcation line between the physician and the physician assistant is not just blurred. It has disappeared. Medical care is now a continuum. The new professionals are playing an increasing role nationally and internationally. Their arrival is changing the face of health care. They are here to stay.

Podiatric surgeons

A similar development has taken place in one area of surgery. The podiatric surgeon (PS), not to be confused with the paediatric surgeon, is a non-medical specialist who is qualified to diagnose and treat disorders of the foot, ankle and related structures. This involves invasive digital and foot surgery, triple arthrodeses, ankle stabilization and Achilles tendon repair. Regulations vary in different countries, but the podiatrist, with advanced training in surgery, may have prescribing rights and privileges, which can include schedule 4 drugs, analgesics and steroids. The PS may also refer patients for X-rays, scans and images. In the UK, highly qualified podiatrists can be appointed to consultant podiatric surgical posts in the NHS.

The older title 'chiropodist' is falling into disuse, but the new nomenclature, podiatric surgeon, has been criticized in some medical circles (especially in orthopaedics) because it may mislead lay people into thinking the PS is medically qualified and regulated by the Royal Colleges. Yet the PS is well trained. In the US, first year classes often overlap with the medical school curriculum. Thereafter the training programme is becoming more directed to disorders of the foot, which is not dissimilar to the focused training of dental surgeons – the 'dentalization' of the foot. Is this a way forward for training in the surgical sub-specialties? Many may disagree, but the trend is evident. The future is already here.

References

1. Crompton S. Learn to trust me, I'm a chemist. Body and Soul. *The Times*, 27 July 2010.
2. Rovner J. Midlevel providers fill primary care doctors' shoes. *National Public Radio*, USA, 27 August 2010.
3. Reynolds T. Medical care practitioners: a necessary import? *Student BMJ* 2006; **14**: 309–52.

CHAPTER 19

Alternative medicine

It is curious that at a time when there is a demand for evidence-based medicine, alternative practitioners, who mostly refuse to have their claims scientifically tested, not only survive, but proliferate and prosper.

Conventional medicine continues to be challenged by alternative medicine. Alternative medicine covers a wide range of largely untested and unregulated remedies. These include neuropathy, herbalism, meditation, reflexology, hypnotherapy, chiropractic, acupuncture, spiritualism, colour therapy, and many other activities.

Chapter summary
- Complementary medicine
- Alternative therapy
- Shamans
- Scientific scrutiny
- Political ambivalence
- Evidence
- Public scepticism
- Music therapy

Complementary medicine

The terms 'complementary', 'holistic' and 'integrated' medicine combine one of these modalities with conventional therapy. A common example is the addition of aromatherapy using floral fragrances following surgery.

Probably most proponents of alternative medicine would first consult an orthodox physician if they developed a significant illness, subsequently adding complementary therapy. Even such a prominent advocate of alternative therapy as Prince Charles has sought conventional treatment on several occasions, including excising a skin lesion, dealing with a polo injury and an inguinal hernia. It may be that he later added herbal remedies to hasten his recovery.

Alternative therapy

Alternative practitioners frequently use the straw man argument to attack the orthodox approach. They misrepresent their opponents' position by creating an illusion, and then refute it.

It is important to distinguish between rogues, charlatans and quacks who shamelessly exploit the sick for financial gain, and those who earnestly believe in quaint remedies for relatively harmless ailments. Some of their beliefs may sound bizarre. For instance, colour therapists believe that colour is a form of energy, and that different colours represent different areas of the body in different states, known as cha.

In the USA, there is considerable interest in detoxing and deep cleansing. According to Spa Finding, a consumer resource for spa information, enquiries in 2009 were up 50% on 2007. One of the more intriguing aspects is the popularity of detox foot pads, which promise to suck out the toxins from your body, via the lymph channels, to the soles of your feet.

Probably, most alternative practitioners deal in the grey areas of back pain, neurasthenia, headaches and lethargy. Even so, all of these complaints can signify the early onset of serious underlying conditions, including metastatic cancer.

There are many reasons why alternative medicine has received widespread support. These include the following:

1. Scientific advances have created unrealistic expectations. The failure of conventional medicine to cure every malady has led some to explore other avenues.

2. There is also the suspicion that orthodox medicine is biased and conservative. This was often exemplified in the past by the medical hierarchy's failure to recognize important advances. One instance already mentioned, which haunts the medical profession, was the shameful derision heaped on Ignaz Semmelweiss in Vienna. This tragic doctor was driven insane trying to persuade obstetricians to wash their hands before delivering infants.

3. Alternative practitioners also quote anecdotal cases and testimonials of cures. Many of these may have been placebo responses. They also include, however, occasional long-term survivals of patients who had 'been given six months to live'. Undoubtedly, some of these cases are factual. But they also occur in conventional medicine. During my career, I had one young man, a rugby player with testicular cancer, who had widespread lung metastases. He had a spontaneous remission and made a complete recovery without any form of treatment. Testicular cancer, to be fair, is an unusual germ cell malignancy that often responds dramatically to treatment; witness the remarkable recovery of the cyclist Lance Armstrong, who had advanced disease, yet went on to win several Tour de France events.

4. Although science has come a long way, there are still things, and always will be, out there we do not understand, or even dream about. Who could have foreseen the existence of electricity before Faraday, Einthoven, Ohm and others? Consider astrophysicists. When they look out into the universe, they ponder not the stars and planets, but the blackness that enfolds them. There have to be biophysical phenomena, forces, energies, call them what you will, that we still have to unravel. The French physicist Bernard D'Espagnet

believes that quantum theory indicates that truth is ultimately veiled from us. His views prompted this strange remark on the Internet from 'Amy in Virginia':

Science only goes so far, and then it falls short. The fact that a change in the oscillation of one photon can be 'felt' by a 2nd photon miles away, (faster than the speed of light), indicates that the two photons are somehow interconnected. Which means there's an additional dimension.

Some alternative practitioners would claim to be visionaries in this regard.

Shamans

The importance of keeping an open mind on claims that sometimes seem preposterous is illustrated by a story currently in vogue about the Shamans.

Shamanism is a range of quasi magico-religious beliefs that exist worldwide, but are practised mostly in the East, particularly in Mongolia. Shamans claim to work beyond the physical body, and act through a trance as intermediaries between the human and the spiritual worlds. Their practices are in some ways close to spiritualism and witchcraft, without perhaps the sinister elements.

The case in point concerns a boy with autism. His story received widespread publicity in a book entitled: *The Horse Boy: A Father's Miraculous Journey to Heal His Son*, by Rupert Isaacson.[1] Isaacson's son Rowan was autistic, incontinent, uncommunicative, and given to nerve-shattering screeching attacks. No form of therapy relieved his condition. The curious relationship with autism and horses has already been discussed. Rowan had had an affinity for horses. As a last resort, his father took him on a riding trip to Mongolia to see the shamans. One Mongolian shaman said that Rowan had been touched by 'black energy' in his mother's womb, and that it was necessary to extract this negative energy. Several archaic rituals were observed. Miraculously, the boy recovered. The case is well documented. Whether Rowan's improvement will be maintained remains to be seen. At the moment, we know very little about autism, or its genetic or environmental roots. A putative prenatal component may not be completely far-fetched. Indeed, new studies on fetal origins confirm that intra-uterine conditions can profoundly influence adult health patterns, ranging from diabetes to mental illness (see later).

Although the shamans are not associated with the Shaolin monks, they share a common culture. The monks are a group of Chinese Buddhists. Their history dates back centuries. They undergo long and arduous training involving self-sacrifice and meditation. The Shaolin monks are especially renowned for their ability in the martial arts. Having seen them in action through Western eyes, I marvelled at their extraordinary acts of endurance, acrobatics and punishing rituals. Some of their feats seemed impossible. I don't believe in black magic, but there are many things that defy our understanding.

Scientific scrutiny

Marcia Angell and Jerome Kassirer outlined the case against alternative medicine in the *New England Journal of Medicine* some years ago.[2] They noted that what sets alternative medicine apart is that 'it has not been scientifically tested, and its advocates largely deny the need for such testing'. It is based on an ideology that largely ignores biological mechanisms, and, worse, disparages scientific scrutiny.

The most common form of alternative therapy is herbal treatment. The botanical base for this has a natural appeal to many. Most of these remedies are probably innocuous, but others may be harmful. Vitamin supplements were discussed earlier. Most people receive adequate nutrients in their normal diet. Occasionally, there may be a case for vitamin therapy – witness the emerging evidence that B-vitamins may delay dementia. But there are also risks associated with hypervitaminosis. Remarkably, these remedies have been exempted from monitoring by the FDA in the USA, because of powerful lobbying by the 'dietary supplement' industry in 1994. Worldwide, this is a multi-billion dollar commercial enterprise. Even the labelling of foodstuffs has been more scrutinized and regulated. The power of this political approach has also been evident in the success of direct-to-consumer advertising of pharmaceutical drugs on television.

Cynics might argue that the public get what they deserve. In a society that idolizes 'celebrities' like Lady Gaga and Amy Winehouse, one should hardly be surprised.

Angell and Kassirer concluded, 'It is time for the scientific community to stop giving alternative medicine a free ride. There cannot be two kinds of medicine, conventional and alternate.' There is only medicine that works, and medicine that does not work. That covers everything. The pharmaceutical industry has had to recognize this, albeit sometimes reluctantly, and agree to clinical trials.[3] The alternative industry should be compelled to follow suit.

Political ambivalence

In the UK, the government approach to alternative therapy has been labelled 'chaotic' by a distinguished group of scientists. One part of government seeks to endorse unproven or disproved treatments, at the same time as another part makes them illegal. The critical authors noted that an official steering group recommended to the Department of Health that university entry into acupuncture, herbal medicine and traditional Chinese medicine should normally be through a Bachelor's degree with honours. In the same month, new regulations in fair-trading noted one case of unfair practice, 'falsely claiming a product is able to cure illness, dysfunctions or malformations'.

The critics claimed that the Department of Health had consistently failed to grasp the nettle of deciding which treatments work, and which do not. This is the first thing that you want to know about any treatment. They suggested that the question be referred to NICE, as with every other form of treatment.

Evidence

The importance of pursuing sound scientific evidence for obscure clinical conditions is illustrated in the search for the cause of post-viral chronic fatigue syndrome (CFS), or myalgic encephalomyelitis. The historical controversy surrounding the very existence of the disease and its treatment has left health care professionals and patient groups confused and arguing about a possible psychological component. However, research now suggests that there may be a link between a human retrovirus and the elusive CFS.

Public scepticism

It is perhaps not surprising that there is sometimes a degree of confusion and scepticism about certain aspects of public health. For instance, the MMR controversy has had a 'knock-on' effect on whooping cough (pertussis). Afraid of autism, 80% parents in three schools in California signed a 'personal belief exemption' to prevent their children being vaccinated. It has been reported that California is now in the midst of its worst outbreak of whooping cough in half a century. Over 2700 cases were reported in August 2010, eight times the previous year's incidence. Seven of the victims, all infants, have died. Dr Harvey Karp, a paediatrician at UCLA, says the parents' concern is understandable.[4] But, he adds, 'The good news is we have a large body of evidence to show zero association between vaccines and autism.' Tolerance and education are essential ingredients in civilized society.

Music therapy

Music therapy is a form of complementary medicine. It is not an alternative to conventional medicine. Music therapists welcome any attempt to give their specialty a scientific basis, and have been involved in several small clinical trials.

Music evolved early in the animal kingdom, as evidenced by the chorus of sound at sunset in a tropical jungle, or the birdsong everywhere at dawn.

The late Professor John Blacking, an ethnomusicologist, agreed with the composer Percy Grainger that folk music is a universal language. It may be that *Homo sapiens* first communicated with each other through musical sounds, before the development of speech.

Music is one of the performing arts. There is no need to prove that people enjoy music. It has been used to relieve stress in mental illness, and enhance the well-being of patients with physical handicaps and communication disorders. One early advocate of music therapy was an Oxford vicar, the Reverend Robert Burton, in the 17th century. Burton himself was depressed, and wrote of the value of music and dance in his book *The Anatomy of Melancholy*.[5]

There is evidence that music therapy improves the outcome of stroke victims. One study of over 30 patients showed that the experimental group, who listened to pleasant music, had a better motor and emotional response than the control group. In a separate small study of three patients who had impaired visual awareness, known as 'visual neglect', there was a marked response to music. Patients with visual neglect lose their awareness and ability to track objects on the opposite side of the damaged brain. In severe cases, patients may only eat food on one side of their plate, or shave only half of their face. Brain scans confirmed that listening to music activated those areas linked to a positive emotional response. Moreover, this activity was coupled with improvement in the patients' performance of tasks.

Music has always been closely associated with movement, as in the dance. And rhythm has been closely related to heartbeat. The neurologist Dr Michael Swallow has pioneered music therapy in Ireland, and made several studies of its value in Parkinson's disease (PD). A striking relationship between music and movement is seen in this condition. Patients with PD exhibit bradykinesia, a slowing of movement, and have great difficulty in sustaining semi-automatic movements such as walking and arm swinging. Swallow and his colleagues have shown how music can release patients with PD from their 'frozen state'.

Swallow has also written extensively about music and communication disorders; about music, emotion, and memory; and the value of music therapy in trauma. He quotes the Sufi Message of Nazrat Iniyat Khan:

Music is the harmony of the universe in microcosm ... and in man ... chords and discords are to be found in his pulse, his heart beat, his vibration, his rhythm and tone. His health or sickness, his joy or displeasure, show whether his life has music or not.

References

1. Isaacson R. *The Horse Boy: A Father's Miraculous Journey to Heal His Son.* Viking: New York, 2009.
2. Angell M, Kassirer JP. Alternative medicine – the risks of untested and unregulated remedies. Editorial. *New England Journal of Medicine* 1998; **339**: 839–41.
3. Bjelakovic G, Nikolova D, Gluud LL et al. Mortality in randomized trials of antioxidant supplements for primary and secondary prevention: systematic review and meta-analysis. *JAMA* 2007; **297**: 842–57.
4. Karp H. Deadly whooping cough, once wiped out, is back. *National Public Radio (NPR)*, 14 August 2010.
5. Burton R. *The Anatomy of Melancholy.* 1621.

CHAPTER 20

Academic medicine and the scientific quest

Medical practice is based on evidence derived from research. Significant advances have been achieved over the years, especially recently. Every day brings a new finding that has to be assessed, scrutinized and

Chapter summary

• Basic research

then absorbed. These developments have sometimes widened the gap between the patient and the physician. That may be the price of progress.

In an attempt to forecast what lies ahead, the strategy underlying medical research deserves closer examination. Academic physicians and scientists have contributed to the advances, in spite of the difficult task of serving many masters. They have to conduct research and to teach, and many also have a clinical commitment to patients. Often forgotten is the fourth dimension, namely the administrative task of coordinating all this activity, fund raising, public speaking, and serving on multiple committees.

Years ago Hugh Cudlipp, the sometime editorial director of the tabloid *Daily Mirror*, entitled his history of the paper *Publish and Be Damned*. In academic medicine, it could read *Publish or Be Damned!* Unfortunately, this has sometimes led to a proliferation of papers of doubtful merit, even in so-called peer review journals. Gone are the days when Louis de Broglie, the young French physicist, could win a Nobel Prize with a Letter to the Editor of *Nature*. Today, scientists have to compete in the marketplace. This has led to an ego race. One would prefer to see more quality than quantity, more humility and less hubris.

In predicting further advances in times of financial restraint, planning productive medical research is essential. The three areas that have proved most rewarding are fundamental research, epidemiology and clinical trials.

Basic research
Curiosity-driven research

It is almost impossible, by definition, to predict revolutionary discoveries. For, if it were possible, they would not be revolutionary. But, as most scientists are confident that the future holds major surprises in store, Donald Braben, former Head of the Venture Research Unit, proposed that the best strategy is to ensure that research is sufficiently diverse so that future bets are covered – spread betting in fact. Serendipity should be allowed to take its course. This has been called *curiosity-driven research*. Elizabeth Blackburn, the Australian who shared the 2009 Nobel Prize with British and American colleagues for their work on the ageing of chromosomes, says their award is a tribute to the value of discoveries driven by curiosity.

Target-oriented research

It is important to distinguish between research and development. Development is the steady improvement and application of an idea. It is an essential part of the overall strategy, but is unlikely by itself to lead to new and unexpected discoveries. Thus applied research or *target-oriented research* has never paid dividends on the same scale as basic research. Research driven by a technique is also less rewarding, since often the technologist's skill is a solution looking for a problem.

The origins of discovery

All basic medical research overlaps at the fundamental level. Hence, for instance, it is no surprise that significant advances in the understanding of AIDS were made in cancer research laboratories. Sir David Weatherall goes further and adds that molecular biology is unifying medicine into a single discipline. Yet attempts at systemizing and unifying the diverse can sometimes lead to over-simplicity, and cause one to ignore relative differences.

Research into the origins of past medical discoveries reveals that these were mostly unanticipated. The Comroe–Dripps study on the origins of ten major advances in cardiovascular medicine showed that few of the advances came from disease-oriented research.[1] The same is true for the origins of advances in anaesthesia. Again, almost all the advances in diagnostic radiology – the discovery of X-rays, ultrasound, CT scanning, magnetic resonance imaging and radioisotopes – were founded in physics laboratories. Similarly, many cancer research workers admit that we will not unravel the final mystery of malignant growth until we fully understand the nature of normal growth.

Timing

Timing is also important. The technology must be available. Pasteur could not have made his discoveries before Leeuwenhoek developed the microscope. Likewise, when Roentgen discovered X-rays, the mathematical equations underlying the CT scanner were quickly solved by Dr Johann Radon in Vienna in the early 1900s. Around the same time, the horizontal anatomical slices were analysed and documented by Professor Johnson Symington FRS in Belfast. But Godfrey Hounsfield could not make computed tomography a reality until the technology became available 60 years later.

Hounsfield himself is interesting in that his background is unconventional. He came out of the RAF after the war, allegedly without even his O-levels, and went on deservedly to be knighted and win the Nobel Prize in Medicine.

Technology from other fields has also contributed to medicine. Techniques used to monitor the vital signs of astronauts have been applied by scientists at Queen's University, to monitor cardiac patients as they go about their daily tasks, whether it be in the office or on the golf course. This work has been extended at St Mary's Hospital in London, using a digital plaster stuck onto the patient's body. The team at Imperial College London hope to market the monitor for a cost of about £20.

Even mathematics may yet have a role. Take chaos theory. Who knows, a bacon sandwich you ate at Gatwick airport last year may help trigger cancer of the pancreas five years down the road.

Biological life is constrained by the immutable laws of the physical world. Some believe the universe is calibrated for life's existence. Thus, the physicists' quest for the Higgs boson (or 'God particle'), and a theory of everything, may yet impact on the medicine of tomorrow.

Compartmentalization

The original simple divisions and boundaries between physics, chemistry and biology have now expanded enormously. The lack of communication between groups has led to the formation of interdisciplinary groups. Coordination has become a buzz word. Interdisciplinary areas have been defined and given priority funding by research councils. Small is no longer beautiful. Many years ago, Sir Alexander Haddow could say, 'I am convinced that the genuine impulse still comes from individual men and women and their new ideas ... support will be given not only to large institutes, but also to individual scientists in small groups in university departments.'

This view, echoed by Kornberg at the time, is out of fashion today in spite of evidence that the concept is still valid. Genetic fingerprinting, the most significant advance in forensic medicine, was discovered in a small cramped laboratory at the University of Leicester. The same is true for the early work of Sydney Brenner, the Nobel Prize-winning molecular biologist. In his retirement, writing of his early research, he said his first grant application was sketched on the backs of a few sheets of paper. He added, 'I hope readers will enjoy a footnote in that application: It read: *To start we propose to identify every cell in the worm and trace lineages.*'

It remains to be seen whether the wheel will go full circle again, spurred by the administrative zeal for reorganization. As T S Eliot remarked, 'A fool is he who thinks he turns the wheel on which he turns.'

Invisible College

Derek de Solla Price, the scientific historian who developed the Citation Index, said that the structure of knowledge is simpler than we thought. Scientific discoveries are closely linked to each other in the literature. There are about two million papers published each year. Surprisingly, there is no more duplication than there ever was. On average, everything is published twice. This is because it is often easier to do an experiment over again than try to find it in the literature. Curiously, scientists today find it no harder to keep up with their own field than before. They are working out at the edge of an expanding circle of knowledge. Specialties subdivide into new specialties as the circle expands. But, at any one time, scientists work in an 'invisible college' of about 200 people. Roughly speaking, on average, most write one *significant* paper a year and read one paper a day. To do so, they have to take into account the work of about 200–300 other people to produce their own material. Occasionally, a new technique enables an important piece to be fitted into the jigsaw, and other pieces follow easily. Breakthroughs are thus often a matter of luck and timing. Price says, for instance, that if Einstein, or Watson and Crick, hadn't made their discoveries, others would have done so within the decade.

Plagiarism

It is important to distinguish between building on the work of previous scientists and plagiarism. Sometimes, research workers are aware of earlier contributions, and acknowledge them; sometimes they are unaware. Edward Jenner probably did not know that others had observed that cowpox infection often conferred a degree of immunity to smallpox.

By all accounts, however, Isaac Newton was an irascible man. His dispute with Leibniz has been described by Stephen Hawking. Both Newton and Leibniz discovered calculus independently. Yet Newton unfairly accused Leibniz of plagiarism, and ridiculed him mercilessly. On the other hand, Einstein would probably have known about *Fitzgerald contraction*. The concept anticipated one aspect of relativity, and was proposed in Dublin by George Francis Fitzgerald in the 19th century. But no one has ever accused Einstein of plagiarism. Watson and Crick, however, were criticized for not giving sufficient recognition to the work of Rosalind Franklin. And Charles Darwin has been accused of pilfering Alfred Russell Wallace's ideas, although most historians refute this allegation. Again, Sir Richard Doll was probably unaware that an association between smoking and cancer had been made in Germany in the 1930s. Banting and Best were certainly unaware that Paulescu in Romania had earlier discovered a compound identical to insulin.

Most remarkably, Alexander Fleming was not the first to discover the value of penicillin, although again there is no question of plagiarism. Ernest Duchesne, a French army physician in the 19th century, had observed the action of *Penicillum glaucum* on the organism *Escherichia coli*. Duchesne made his discovery having noted that Arab stable boys kept their saddles in the dark, to encourage mould to grow, which in turn healed saddle sores on horses. The Institute Pasteur did not even acknowledge Duchesne's dissertation. Even earlier, in 1875, the Irish physicist John Tyndall demonstrated the antibacterial action of penicillin. He presented his findings to the Royal Society. But neither Duchesne nor Tyndall had the opportunity to follow up their discoveries.

There has always been a race to be first in print with a new idea, but plagiarism is uncommon and most of the time the race is open and fair. Meanwhile, one might wonder what important scientific discoveries have already been made, yet overlooked and consigned to a bottom drawer somewhere.

Ideas

The philosopher Polanyi offered the following definition: *'Research is the intuition of rationality in nature, rather than a collection of observations and facts.'* The facts, of course, are essential, but the intuition is derived from curiosity. Ideas emerge from educated and informed discussion, and careful reflection. They require a free and creative environment and time for debate. An atmosphere of insecurity, far from 'focusing the mind marvellously', makes one concentrate on scheming for survival. Necessity may be the mother of invention, but adversity is not the father of discovery. Kenneth Clark in his Opus Magnus *Civilisation*, noted that Art flourishes in a relaxed era and in times of plenty. The same may be true of Science.

Thought experiments

Einstein and Newton did not pioneer thought experiments, but they were perhaps the best-known exponents. The concept in the biological sciences of theoretical medicine has not yet been fully developed. Theoretical concepts allow models to be constructed and ideas to be tested. Only when they have been tested experimentally are they accepted in the scientific marketplace. And incidentally, only experimentally proven findings qualify for Nobel laureates. If the theories do not work, they must be discarded.

Denis Burkitt likened progress in science to a happy marriage. You must admit when you are wrong. A former medical Dean at Queen's University, Ian Roddie, said that there should be a journal awarding credit for negative results. Scientists need to be adaptable and prepared to modify their plans if results point in a different direction. One may have a compass and a general sense of direction in medical research, but there are no charts that map out the future.

Time

Probing the innermost secrets of nature requires time, concentration and patience. The late Richard Feynman, the Nobel Prize-winning theoretical physicist, emphasized the importance of taking adequate time to do research. The following is a short transcript I made of a broadcast interview I heard him give on the BBC Television programme *Horizon*:

> *To do the sort of thing I am talking about, you need absolute solid lengths of time. It's like constructing a house of cards. When you are putting the cards together on top of each other, you must not shake them. If you forget one of them, the whole thing collapses again. You don't know how you got there. And you have to build them up again. And if you are interrupted, you forget half the idea of how the cards went*

together. Your cards being different parts of ideas of different kinds that have to go together to build up the total concept, the complete structure. You put it all together. It's quite a tower. And it's easy to slip. And it needs a lot of concentration, that is solid time to think.

Feynman scoffed at the administrative role. He would not allow his train of thought to be interrupted by committee work. He famously said of administration, 'Let George do it'. Few can afford this luxury. Professors and academic staff, encumbered with multi-tasking, still have to convince others of the value of their work.

Questions

The frequent interruptions in a busy clinician's life are not the only hazard in medical research. Kornberg and Sackett have drawn attention to the importance of asking the right questions. Questions need to be logically well founded. It is the essence of scientific discipline to ask simple, discrete, clear and well-defined questions. They must then be addressed effectively if useful results are to be obtained. Obviously, one doesn't ask imponderable questions such as 'What is the cure for cancer?' But even at the simple level, phrases such as 'disease-free interval' and 'disease-free survival' have sometimes been confused. Sloppy thinking will lead to sloppy results.

Measurement

Measurement also matters. It is necessary to put numbers on one's findings, otherwise, as Kelvin noted, 'our knowledge is of an unsatisfactory kind'. The collection of data calls for meticulous attention to detail if it is to be meaningful. Sir Thomas Symington noted that false theories advance science, but false facts retard it. Feynman added his concern about the accumulation of pseudoscientific data:

Experts who fool themselves. They don't do scientific work. They follow the forms. But they don't discover fundamental particles or define Laws of Nature. They don't realize how difficult it is to really get to know something. How careful you have to be about checking the experiments. How easy it is to make mistakes and fool yourself.

Many clinical trials have produced contradictory results because of such problems.

Innovation

Braben emphasized that it is not sufficient to have an expansive idea in medical research. Grandiose plans are not at a premium. There should be credibility and some prospect, however distant, of eventual innovation. Ideas therefore need to be realistic. Realism may be defined as modest optimism in research. Everyone can contribute to the slow accumulation of knowledge. The development of modern medicine owes much to the quiet painstaking observations of hundreds of physicians over the years. The eponyms that a number of diseases carry in medicine bear credit to many of these doctors. Yet the public should not expect too much from research. Overnight breakthroughs are rare, and usually follow years of patient slog. Targets should be set within the measurable space of a man's lifetime. Kornberg has noted that the clinical scientist fails when he lets problems choose and dominate him, rather than the reverse. He recommends selecting one, just one, intriguing question and grappling with it for as long as it takes. The need to focus sharply on a single problem over a long space of time is central to Kornberg's scientific philosophy. By the same token, he adds that one should avoid undertaking excessively complex problems in a gamble for quick payoffs.

Dr Earl Green, the former Director of the Jackson Laboratories in Bar Harbor, Maine, told me that, just before he retired, he toured the facility to say goodbye to his colleagues. He came to one laboratory where two scientists had been working for many years on the problem of how one cell divides into two. He asked them how they were getting on with the project. They replied, 'We are not quite ready to start yet. We are still trying to devise a satisfactory medium in which to isolate the mouse zygote'!

In the end, scientific success, like success in other areas of life, flows from the individual and his enthusiasm. As Oscar Wilde opined, it is personalities, not principles, that shape the age. The lifestyle guru Wayne Dyer adds, it requires passion.

Funding

Research is expensive, and someone has to pay for it. Financial support for basic research must be given as an Act of Faith. It is not derived from a Law of Economics. Sir James Black, another Nobel Laureate, says his chief worry is that there is no room for Friday afternoon experiments. Projects must be conventional. He says that the work he did many years ago on beta-blockers would probably not be funded today.

There is also the political dimension. Elizabeth Blackburn is an outspoken research worker. She was fired in 2004 from President George W Bush's Council on Bioethics, in what many scientists believed was her criticism of his policy on human embryonic stem cell research. The Bush advisors had no reason to believe that the work she had already done would eventually lead to a Nobel Award. One of the first decisions of the Obama administration was to reverse the decision on stem cell research.

Publication

It may be that many useful scientific ideas have never been published, because they have been rejected, unwritten or consigned to the bottom drawer. Thomas Harriot is one example. He was an early astronomer who made many observations, including Saturn's rings, Jupiter's position, and sunspots. In July 1609, he made an intricate map of the Moon's surface, craters and seas, four months before Galileo's astronomical recordings were made. But, unlike Galileo, who thrived on publicity, and needed money, Harriot was a self-effacing nobleman who never saw the need to publish his work.[2] If he had done so, he might have been a household name.

An idea needs to be marketed. Until it is tested, there is no way of knowing its true worth. If it isn't published, it doesn't exist. There is an added benefit in writing up the findings. It forces the scientist to clarify his thoughts. The philosopher Wittgenstein put it aptly: 'What can be said, can be said clearly. Whereof one cannot speak, one must be silent.' I would add, a great idea embodied in a single sentence is the goal. Ohm's law is a case in point, or Darwin's theory of evolution. One wit summed it up: *Eschew obscurantism.*

References

1. Comroe Jr JH, Dripps RD. Scientific basis for the support of biomedical science. *Science* 1976; **192**: 105–11.
2. Devlin H. Revealed: the Englishman who made his first foray into space before Galileo. *The Times*, 24 July 2009.

CHAPTER 21

Epidemiology and uncertainty in medicine

Bedside epidemiology

Chapter summary
- Bedside epidemiology
- The clinical principle of uncertainty

The role of laboratory research is self-evident. But many of the more immediate problems in medicine have been solved not in the laboratory, but by epidemiology. Medical science is often based on probability rather than certainty. This is true of both epidemiology and clinical trials.

Epidemiology begins and ends at the bedside. Bedside epidemiology has been something of a Cinderella in medicine. Yet it is true that public health measures did more to combat cholera than antibiotics. And it is generally agreed that one of the greatest discoveries in cancer research over the past 60 years has been establishing the link between smoking and lung cancer. Remarkably, the epidemiologists who made the discovery, Richard Doll, Bradford Hill and Court Brown, were not recognized by the Nobel Committee. Epidemiology is outside the terms of the Nobel Awards. Moreover, apart from lung cancer, smoking has been linked with a number of other malignancies, and with sudden cardiac death, emphysema and a miscellaneous group of conditions.

Many other advances have been made in epidemiology, ranging from identifying a link between AIDS and intravenous drug use to the association between malignant melanoma, skin cancer and solar radiation.

Epidemiological research requires observation, curiosity and patience. It often requires years to uncover new features. It also requires close scrutiny, to avoid faulty reasoning. The ancients were aware of this. The Latin phrase *post hoc ergo propter hoc*, meaning 'after this, therefore because of this', is a common logical fallacy: *A* occurred, then *B* occurred; therefore, *A* caused *B*. Eighty percent of patients who developed breast cancer were in the supermarket last week; therefore, the supermarket is a dangerous place to visit. And there are many other pitfalls and biases discussed earlier.

The need for close liaison between the clinician, the laboratory worker, the epidemiologist and the statistician has now been recognized. Increasingly, the molecular biologist is telling the epidemiologist where to look.

The clinical principle of uncertainty

Clinical trials are essential for clinical progress. If a new drug is introduced and the effects are dramatic, there is little need for prolonged multicentre trials. It is a penicillin effect. But most of the time this is not the case. Unfortunately, improvements in therapy are often small. Marginal differences in survival can then only be detected by very large trials. This creates its own problems. For instance, a comprehensive study on breast cancer, entitled 'Combinant adjuvant chemotherapy for node positive breast cancer', studied 2628 patients, of whom 1229 fulfilled the criteria essential to the study. To obtain this number of patients, the study involved eight countries on three continents with 189 contributors. The 189 authors had to be listed in a special appendix in the publication. A small difference was detected. One colleague remarked 'little differences matter little'. They do, of course, matter for those few patients – but only if the differences are real and can be relied on.

In another study, of myocardial infarction, contradictory results were obtained between an overview of earlier trials and a subsequent mega-trial or meta-analysis. The benefits of nitrates and magnesium, which had reduced mortality by 50% in earlier trials, disappeared completely in the mega-trial. The additional patients who survived in the earlier trials were dismissed as statistical pawns in the random analysis. An alternative explanation might be that 'personalization' of treatment, or environmental factors in subgroups, may have enhanced their survival. Such factors may not only be unknown, they may be unknowable.

In the mega-trial, tens of thousands of patients, managed by several thousand doctors, were seen in 32 countries spread over five continents. The hope was that the differences would be smoothed out in the meta-analysis. It is difficult to accept that quality control was evenly sustained throughout such a massive undertaking.

As mentioned earlier by Feynman, experts can fool themselves. They don't realize how difficult it is to really get to know something. Clinicians who have been involved in trials over decades are fully aware not only of the vast number of clinical variables from patient to patient, but also the difficulty of obtaining meaningful scientific data in busy hospital departments, overwhelmed with paperwork and coping with the daily problems of sick patients and anxious relatives. This is compounded when trials are outsourced to the Third World. India is not a Third World country, but the scandal involving the death of 49 babies in a drug trial in India has already been mentioned. Oversight is not only lax, it is often non-existent. So, although larger numbers theoretically enable one to detect smaller statistical differences, paradoxically this is offset by the deterioration in quality control.

There is also the problem of informed consent. In the USA, many patients who have been fully informed are refusing to enter trials. Informed consent has become a contradiction in terms. In addition, there is a 'Heisenberg effect'. The act of informing a patient may affect the patient and disturb the study. Once patients have been informed, trials can no longer be blind. If one arm of a trial consists of a harmless placebo, such as glucose, there are no side effects, whereas the active arm will almost always have some unwanted effect that is quickly noted.

Another problem relates to meta-analysis. These studies, which sometimes combine the results of dozens of separate trials, rely on published work. As mentioned earlier, negative studies are often not published. This publication bias is called the 'file drawer effect', where negative studies are buried and end up in the bin, rather than the literature. There is the added problem of 'wish bias', the conscious or unconscious overestimation of effects in non-blinded studies. Again, the extent to which some pharmaceutical companies influence the design and outcome of trials is a major cause for concern. Equally, the conflict of interest of many clinicians conducting the trials has been deplored.

For all these reasons, there is inevitably a lower limit below which one cannot detect differences between two arms of a clinical trial. The statistical noise obscures the result. So progress in this field is often two steps forward, and one step back.

CHAPTER 22

New medicine

The results of scientific endeavour have created a new wave of research topics. These include advances in genetics, epigenetics, stem cells, antisense therapy, nanoparticles and molecular pathology. The impact of these discoveries is radically changing the face of medicine.

Many of these developments involve reductionism, sometimes referred to as downward causation. This involves reducing a complex system, in this case biology, into its component parts, and then studying these in isolation. Philosophers argue that such systems are not necessarily the sums of their parts. But the trend in biological research persists.

Genetic counselling

It was Gregor Mendel, a monk in the Abbey of St Thomas in Brno (of which he later became Abbott), who first formulated the laws of inheritance. Sadly, his work was not fully recognized during his lifetime, and his seminal paper in *Proceedings of the Natural History Society of Brunn* in 1865, was hardly cited during his career. It was William Bateson of Cambridge, England, who later championed Mendel, and coined the term 'genetics'.

Mendel studied almost 30,000 pea plants and set the stage for the classic description of dominant, recessive, and X-linked modes of inheritance, later expanded to include multifactorial disorders.

Today genetic counsellors still use Mendel's laws to advise prospective parents, on the basis of their family history, about the chances of their offspring developing a variety of disorders. These range from simple conditions such as colour blindness

Chapter summary

- Genetic counselling
- Gene therapy
- Antisense therapy
- The central dogma
- The Weismann principle
- Nature/nurture and epigenetics
- Monoclonal antibodies
- Oncogenes
- Stem cell research
- Angiogenesis
- Nanomedicine
- Biogenesis
- Creating artificial life

to more serious diseases such as haemophilia, cystic fibrosis, Huntington's disease, muscular dystrophy and achondroplasia.

Following the discovery of DNA, molecular genetics refined Mendel's work. This culminated in mapping the entire human genome, the molecular equivalent of *Gray's Anatomy*. Today, many rogue genes have been isolated in a variety of diseases. In these cases, a simple test has enabled counsellors to discuss with patients who carry the affected gene their various options. Common examples include the *BRCA1* gene in breast cancer and the gene responsible for hereditary cardiomyopathy. Patients at very high risk can then decide whether to undergo say, bilateral mastectomy to eliminate the probability of developing breast cancer. Lesser genetic defects also continue to be identified. For instance, the *BAK* gene causes deafness in elderly patients, destroying the hair cells in the inner ear. The hope is that this gene can also be excised or disabled, halting the onset of deafness.

Testing for a single-gene disease is relatively straightforward. But multigene disorders are more complex, and testing for them seems premature. Detailed genetic profiling is still some distance away, yet firms are offering this facility at costs between £500 and £800. In a *Sunday Times* inquiry published in September 2008, Nic Fleming, an investigative journalist, had his own DNA samples tested by three different companies.[1] According to his report, the results gave 'widely divergent and inaccurate predictions of his chances of developing serious diseases'. He concluded that these conflicting results could either give misleading assurances or cause needless anxiety. Christine Patch of Guy's Hospital, a member of the Human Genetics Commission, is quoted as saying, 'these companies are identifying gene types correctly', but the interpretation of the variants is 'still work in progress'.

Nonetheless, commercial firms will probably continue to offer genetic profiling to those who wish to pay for it. Once again, science is bypassing the doctor and going directly to the consumer. As the idiom goes, the physician is left 'piggy in the middle'.

Genetic predictions will become more refined in time. But, as with any statistical evaluation, one can never be certain of the outcome. Even though the chance of developing a certain condition is assessed as extremely high, there is always the interplay of nature and nurture.

The ethical implications of this work are among the more important facing society today. Not least is whether such information should be made available to, say, life insurance carriers. At present, failure to disclose relevant medical information could render policies null and void. This is no longer the exclusive domain of the medical profession. It now involves a range of professionals and others, including lawyers, the clergy, politicians, psychologists and insurance executives.

Nonetheless, there is one area where genetic research is advancing rapidly. That is in mapping the genetic code of individual cancers.[2] James Watson summed it up: 'Cancer is a disease of the DNA.' Mapping has already been achieved in a few patients. The genetic chart of a 55-year-old man with lung cancer revealed 22,910 mutations, mostly due to smoking. In a second case, 33,345 mutations were found in a 43-year-old man with malignant melanoma, probably due to ultraviolet solar exposure. The findings raise the possibility of targeting genetic damage with designer drugs tailored for individual patients, depending on their cancer profile. This would be a Herculean task, if it meant personalizing treatment for every patient. But it is thought that, out of thousands of damaged genes, common errors will be shared between groups of patients, permitting specific drugs to be designed for these cases (see Colour Plate 4).

This new field is known as pharmacogenomics. Francis Collins, who led the Human Genome Project, predicts that bespoke genetic health care will become available in the next decade, if not sooner.[3] He estimates that the cost of genetic sequencing for an individual may eventually drop from the present $10,000 to $1000.

Gene therapy

Although everyone carries a handful of defective genes, genetic disorders are fortunately relatively uncommon. This is because chromosomes come in pairs, and we all carry a copy of most genes on the opposing chromosome. If one gene is damaged, the other usually covers the defect. Exceptions to this occur if the damaged gene is so strong or dominant that it overcomes the normal counterpart. Also, since males have only one X chromosome, if the defective gene is on this chromosome, there is no corresponding normal gene (this is the case in X-linked disorders such as haemophilia).

Genetic disorders can be passed down from one generation to another. Cystic fibrosis is an example. Or the genetic damage can be acquired as a result of a mutation. Leukaemia induced by radiation would be an example.

Gene therapy uses genes to prevent or treat such disorders. Several methods have been tried. The most common technique inserts a normal gene into the genome to replace the damaged gene. Alternatively, an abnormal gene can be swapped with a normal gene. Thirdly, the abnormal gene may be repaired by reverse mutation. In another technique, the genetic switch may be altered to turn the function of the gene on or off.

To achieve these results, a vector is sometimes used to carry the gene or the repair kit into the cellular domain. The most commonly used vector is a virus. The virus then unloads its spare part into the damaged zone. Non-viral methods have also been investigated. These techniques are moving forward rapidly, but are still largely in the domain of the research laboratory. Some preliminary encouraging results have been obtained treating 'Lorenzo's Oil' brain disease, a genetic disorder known as adrenoleukodystrophy (ALD). The approach uses a virus to carry a working copy of the gene that is faulty in ALD (the *ABCD1* gene) into the patient, correcting the defect.

Laboratory tests at Leeds University in England have shown how proteins can be added to a virus in order to enable it to recognize unique markers on the surface of tumours. Dr John Chester, who led the study, said the virus could then deliver genes to cancer cells.[4] These genes can make the cancer more sensitive to drugs; 'suicide' genes can be introduced, or missing or defective genes that cause cancer can be replaced.

In a separate trial,[5] damaged lungs have been repaired, making them fit for transplant. About 80% of donor lungs are unsuitable for transplant, because of damage following brain death. The new technique uses an adenovirus vector, carrying an added interleukin-10 (IL-10) gene, which is inserted into the damaged lungs. The gene 'turbocharges' each cell to manufacture anti-inflammatory proteins in its own IL-10 factory. These in turn repair the damaged lungs, making them suitable for transplant. Nearly 10,000 people are waiting for life-saving transplants. The hope is that the new technique can be extended to other damaged donor organs.[6]

Antisense therapy

Antisense therapy is a similar form of treatment. Strictly speaking, it is not gene therapy, but it is genetically mediated. Although genes carry the genetic information in their DNA, it is the proteins they instruct that carry out the orders. This is done through messenger RNA, which is a single-stranded molecule (as opposed to the double-helix DNA). This single-stranded structure can sometimes be elegantly blocked by a complementary protein, called an antisense protein.

Gene therapy and antisense therapy have been tried on a number of disorders. These include two of the most intransigent cancers: malignant melanoma and pancreatic cancer. So far, only limited success has been obtained, but it is hoped that this two-pronged approach will yield future dividends.

The central dogma

Any discussion of gene therapy must take account of the central dogma of molecular biology. This states that information only travels in one direction, from DNA to RNA to protein. The subsequent discovery of reverse transcriptase, by Howard Temin and David Baltimore, showed that the reverse is possible. It was as if the workers were telling the foreman what to do, and where to go! The discovery led to the identification of retroviruses, notably HIV, the cause of AIDS.

The Weismann principle

A similar principle to the central dogma, the Weismann principle, has also been challenged. The Weismann principle states that hereditary information only flows from germline cells to body cells, and never the reverse. In other words, somatic to germline feedback is impossible. There is now evidence that the Weismann barrier is permeable, and that genes can be passed horizontally between species.[7] This is due to the 'cut-and-paste' action of certain viruses. Characteristics acquired during an organism's lifetime could thus be inherited. It raises the worrying possibility that gene therapy could alter the genetics of the human species, rather than the individual patient.

This has reopened the controversial Lamarckian dispute. Lamarck believed in the inheritance of acquired characteristics. In the West, he was ridiculed as a heretic. In Russia, however, his ideas were hailed by Lysenko, the director of Soviet biology under Stalin. Lysenko approved of Lamarckism, noting that political changes imposed on society could be inherited. Scientists were expected to conform to the Marxian philosophy of dialectical materialism. Those who disagreed were sent to the gulags or disappeared. The debate is a disturbing reminder of the conflict that sometimes arises between science and society. It also demonstrates that dogma has no place in the laboratory.

Nature/nurture and epigenetics

The long-running discussion on whether hereditary or environment plays a greater role in determining or shaping an individual's behaviour, the nature/nurture debate, now has a scientific base. It is called epigenetics: *epi* (Greek 'over' or 'above') genetics.

Epigenetics is the study of heritable changes in gene function that do not change DNA sequence, but rather provide an 'extra' layer of translational control that regulates how genes are expressed.

The human genome consists of 23,000 genes that must be switched on to be expressed in specific cells at precise times. It is now recognized that much of the 'junk DNA' previously thought to have no important function may turn genes on and off. These switches are controlled by the addition of a methyl group to DNA, known as DNA methylation. This fluctuates in response to environmental agents such as diet, smoking and viruses.

Epigenetics has thus shown how non-genetic factors can cause an organism to express itself or behave differently. It is also involved in normal morphogenesis, whereby totipotential cells become pluripotential cells in the embryo, and in turn become fully differentiated cells in different organs.

Monoclonal antibodies

Some years ago, I noted that infants not only inherit passive immunity to infection from their mothers during the first year of life, they also inherit immunity to cancer.[8] This immunity declines in older children, who are prone to develop the cancers and leukaemias of childhood. The protective effect appears to be due to maternal antibodies. The finding anticipated a possible role for antibodies in malignant disease.

One of the first to investigate immunotherapy was Dr William Coley, a New York surgeon at the end of the 19th century. He reported a case of spontaneous tumour regression in a patient following an attack of erysipelas. Coley then prepared a vaccine out of dead streptococcus bacteria, and injected it into an abdominal tumour in a teenage boy. The lad had a massive immunological reaction with fever, and the tumour began to regress. Other physicians reported similar responses. But the results were not sustained, and the treatment fell into disuse. For years, immunotherapy proved disappointing. This was probably because immunology is based on the concept of self and non-self. And as cancer cells are essentially part of self, they are not easily rejected. Nevertheless, malignant cells are abnormal in several ways and contain unusual antigens on their cell surface receptors. It is these flawed receptors that are now targeted by monoclonal antibodies.

Two naturally occurring immunological features have been adapted to create clusters of monoclonal antibodies in the laboratory. First, when the body is invaded by infection, the immune system responds to the foreign antigen with a shotgun response, producing a range of polyclonal antibodies. Second, a malignant disease of plasma cells in the bone marrow, known as multiple myeloma, can produce a shower of antibodies from a single clone.

The production of monoclonal antibodies has gone through several developmental stages. The first method involved injecting a laboratory mouse to produce murine antibodies. These were then fused with immortalized cells from multiple myeloma, forming a hybridoma, producing large quantities of monoclonal antibodies. Unfortunately, innate differences between the mouse and human resulted in early problems, including allergic reactions. A more refined method uses transgenic mice, transferring the human immunoglobulin into the neutral mouse genome. The mouse is then vaccinated with the specific antigen, producing the required human monoclonal antibody.

Monoclonal antibodies have been applied for both diagnostic and therapeutic purposes. In diagnosis, they can be used to detect small quantities of a given substance in a western blot test or an immunofluorescence test. They can also be used to detect the presence of drugs in the system, or to diagnose pregnancy or AIDS. Furthermore, they are being tested as tumour markers in diagnosing or monitoring disease response or progression.

The therapeutic use of monoclonal antibodies has expanded enormously. At present, over a score of compounds have been created, and are being used routinely or are being tested in clinical trials. One of the first was the discovery that the ErbB2 receptor (also known as HER2/neu), in about 30% of cases of breast cancer, could be blocked by the monoclonal antibody trastuzumab (Herceptin), retarding the progression of the disease.

Most of the trials have involved malignant disease, but several other conditions have been targeted, including rheumatoid arthritis, transplant rejection, macular degeneration and haemoglobinuria. Not surprisingly, there has been a scramble by pharmaceutical companies to produce these remarkable new designer drugs.

Oncogenes

One of the most intriguing advances in medicine is the discovery that every living cell in the human body contains all the information in its molecular switchboard to make an entire human being. In mature cells, most of this information is switched off, and only the specialized features of the particular organ are activated.

In cancer, the genetic switches – the oncogenes and tumour suppressor genes – that trigger or block malignant transformation have been intensively studied, together with the complex signal transduction pathways. This work is proceeding at a feverish pace.

Stem cell research

Cellular growth begins with conception. Following this initial event, the fertilized egg rapidly divides into a blastocyst, containing *totipotential* stem cells in a matter of a few days. As these embryonic stem cells continue to divide, each new cell has the potential either to continue as an adult stem cell or to differentiate into a specialized cell, such as a blood cell, a muscle cell, a heart cell, and so on.

Embryonic stem cells are therefore extremely useful in research. They can be manipulated to become specialized cells to repair tissues that have been damaged by injury or disease.

Inevitably, this work is highly controversial, in that it is argued that experimenting with embryonic cells is tampering with the origin of life itself.

There is less controversy, however, regarding the use of adult stem cells, which reside in the bone marrow, since these cells have already fulfilled their developmental role. Unfortunately, adult stem cells are more difficult to culture in sufficient numbers to be useful. However, it has recently been possible to take adult *skin* cells, reverse the process of differentiation, and take the cells back to their embryonic state. They can then be reprogrammed and persuaded to develop into any of the several hundred cell types in the body.

The Chinese Academy of Sciences has taken these reprogrammed cells, known as induced pluripotent stem cells (iPS), one step further. Previously, iPS cells could be persuaded to turn into a variety of cells, but not into a living creature. Before that, cloning had only been achieved by inserting DNA from an adult cell into an empty egg. The Chinese work has enabled iPS cells in a mouse to be turned into a living clone.

All of these developments raise possibilities in regenerative medicine. For instance, in one experiment, the heart of a rat was stripped of its cellular material and then repopulated with cells from the organ of another decellurized rat. It is foreseen that this may lead to retooling, of say the human cadaver heart for repair work in patients with cardiac disease.

Developing this technique involves taking, say, a donor heart valve, and then stripping its cells using a cocktail of enzymes and detergents. The inert scaffold is then inserted and is no longer rejected by the host's immune system. The body then takes over and repopulates the scaffold.

Beyond organ building, it is envisaged that it may be possible to persuade damaged nerve fibres to regenerate along fine tubes in cases of paraplegia. Another intriguing possibility is the proposal to create artificial glands to test new drugs, rather than using tissue cultures or animal experiments.

Already, stem cell studies have offered hope in repairing damaged hearts. Trials are underway at Bart's Hospital and University College Hospital, London, injecting stem cells directly into heart attack victims. Early results are encouraging. Again, as mentioned earlier, stem cells have been used in Southampton, in lieu of prostheses, in hip replacement surgery. The acetabulum cavity was filled with stem cells mixed with 'cleaned' bone from another patient. In a more remarkable case, also discussed earlier, a young Spanish woman with tuberculosis of the trachea had a donor windpipe cleaned from a dead patient, used as a scaffold, and then repopulated with the patient's own stem cells. This procedure has now been used on several patients where the stem cells were grown both in the laboratory and in the body.

In another advance, a technique has been developed to avoid searching for matched donor bone marrow transplants. The present approach to treating some diseases, such as leukaemia, involves killing off malignant marrow cells and replacing them with cells from a healthy matched donor. Matched donors are difficult to find. The new technique takes stem cells from the umbilical cord of newborn infants, which have not yet acquired immune characteristics. These primitive cells are then manipulated and multiplied in the laboratory. They can then be used to treat adult patients, without the danger of GVH (graft versus host) reaction.

Professor Colleen Delaney,[9] who, along with a team from the Fred Hutchinson Cancer Research Unit in Seattle, pioneered this work, exclaimed, 'I mean it's amazing. You can take someone else's trash – right when a baby is born you give life to that infant – at the same time you can save the cells from the umbilical cord and give life to someone else who potentially needs life saving treatment.'

This work is proceeding rapidly. Hans Clevers and a team of Dutch and Swedish scientists have found the 'mother of all' skin stem cells, the cell that makes all the other skin cells.[10] These cells have a high level of a gene called *LGR6*.[11] The hope is that this work will dramatically improve the treatment of wounds and burns.

Only a few years ago, Lord Robert Winston, in his Presidential Address to the British Association for the Advancement of Science in 2005, was sceptical about the hype surrounding stem cell research. Since then, the work has moved rapidly. No doubt this research will surge forward in the USA, now that Barak Obama[12] has lifted the eight-year ban on embryonic stem cell studies imposed by the previous Bush administration.[13]

Meanwhile, exaggerated claims have been made on some commercial websites for stem cell therapy. The International Society for Stem Cell Research says patients are being exploited and given false hope.[14] An investigation of 19 companies that promote such therapies found that most make inflated claims about benefits that are not backed by evidence. Moreover, there is often little mention of the risks. One expert, Professor George Daley of Boston Children's Hospital, says these websites are dangerous. The public need to understand how many years of research are required before novel stem cell therapies can be brought to fruition. The direct-to-consumer advertising in North America has been widely deplored. Although this has been regulated to some extent, advertising on the Internet is largely uncontrolled.

At present, only a few stem cell procedures have been officially approved. These include treatments for leukaemia and the management of burns. Another exciting development involves multiple sclerosis. In this, rogue lymphocytes that damage the myelin insulation of nerve sheaths were replaced by new lymphocytes formed from stem cells. These effectively reset the patient's immune system, preventing further damage.

Although this work offers promise for those disabled by chronic conditions, predictions of a rosy future for an ageing population seem premature, if not naive.

We have seen how advances in nuclear physics have been both used and abused. The same may be true for the biological revolution. Spare parts surgery is a splendid goal, but the ethical controversy surrounding stem cell research is understandable.

Creating a chimera, a living organism that incorporates two distinct species in its DNA, is a disturbing concept. It undermines the distinction between humans and animals. Already, hybrid human–cow embryos have been created in the laboratory to enable stem cell studies. The prospect of creating a centaur is grotesque. We will return to this development.

Angiogenesis

Another area of medical research that has received considerable attention is angiogenesis. This is the normal process that induces the growth of blood vessels. It occurs spontaneously in the development of the vascular system in newborn infants. It also helps to repair wound healing by promoting growth from existing blood vessels.

Unfortunately, angiogenesis also occurs pathologically in malignant tumours. Cancer cells release activator proteins that increase vascularization. This enables tumours to metastasize and spread to distant parts of the body.

It is also evident in macular degeneration. In wet macular degeneration, excess growth factor increases the permeability of blood vessels. This releases blood and oedema, and promotes capillary growth in the retina, thereby causing visual deterioration.

On the positive side, angiogenesis has been promoted in cardiovascular disease, using chemical stimulants, such as fibroblast growth factor (FGF), to improve blood flow. Preclinical investigations have had mixed success in cardiac ischaemia and peripheral vascular disease.

The bulk of research, however, has been in malignant disease. Normally, the walls of blood vessels are formed by vascular endothelial cells that only divide every few years. They are only switched on to divide when required. This process is regulated by a balance between activator and inhibitor proteins. Cancer cells upset this balance by releasing excess activator proteins. To prevent this in malignancy, the process can be blocked by angiogenesis inhibitors. Several of these compounds have been developed, including endostatin and bevacizumab (Avastin).

Interestingly, thalidomide, a drug that was used as a sedative in pregnancy decades ago with disastrous results, has found a novel role as an angiogenesis inhibitor in cancer. Formerly, in one of several possible actions, it blocked the growth of blood vessels in the developing limb of the fetus, leading sadly to deformities.[15] In its new role, it inhibits the vascularization and growth of malignant tumours.

Angiogenesis inhibitors are cancerostatic, not cancerocidal. That is, they retard or block the expansion of tumours, but they do not obliterate them. Nonetheless, they are extremely useful. Their mode of action is similar to that of the sulphonamides, the bacteriostatic drugs that predated the bactericidal antibiotics.

Nanomedicine

Any discussion of the future of medicine must consider the rapidly advancing field of nanotechnology. Curiously, the concept is not new. Nanoparticles were used by medieval potters in glazing, to produce lustre on the surface of porcelain and ceramics. Today, nanomedicine is one of the most exciting areas of medical research.

This is the Lilliputian world of molecular manufacturing. Previously the common unit of measurement in the microscopic world was the micrometre or micron (μm). The micrometre is used, for instance, to measure wavelengths at the longer end of the electromagnetic spectrum, in the infrared region. It equals one millionth of a metre. In nanotechnology, the unit of measurement is much smaller, the nanometre (nm). This equals one billionth of a meter. It largely replaces the Ångström unit (Å), which is 0.1 nm. Some tiny bacteria, for instance, measure about 200 nm, the DNA double helix 2 nm and the smallest molecules a fraction of that. Nanotechnology can be considered from a 'top-down' approach or a 'bottom-up' approach. Approaching from the top, nanoparticles are created from larger objects. In the bottom-up method, nanodevices are created from the molecules themselves.

The molecular world obeys the laws of physics, as in the larger world, but quantum and other effects can create unusual phenomena. For instance at the nanolevel, solids can sometimes behave as liquids, and opaque materials can become invisible. Moreover, as particles diminish in size, the geometry changes (see box). The surface area increases compared with the volume. Thus, the contact with the surroundings is greater than with larger objects. This high surface-area-to-volume ratio makes nanoparticles very reactive or catalytically active. Much smaller than living cells, they can easily pass through cell membranes.

Nanogeometry

The circumference of a circle depends on the radius ($2\pi r$), whereas the area depends on the square of the radius (πr^2). Thus, as the radius contracts, the area decreases faster than the circumference.

The same applies to solid objects. The surface area of a sphere is proportional to the square of the radius ($4\pi r^2$), whereas the volume is proportional to the cube ($\frac{1}{3}\pi r^3$). Thus, as the radius contracts, the volume diminishes faster than the surface area.

For example, for a circle:

Radius (r)	Circumference ($2\pi r$)	Area (πr^2)	Ratio of area to circumference ($\frac{1}{2}r$)
3	6π	9π	1.5
2	4π	4π	1
1	2π	π	0.5
$\frac{1}{2}$	π	$\frac{1}{4}\pi$	0.25
$\frac{1}{4}$	$\frac{1}{2}\pi$	$\frac{1}{16}\pi$	0.125
$\frac{1}{6}$	$\frac{1}{3}\pi$	$\frac{1}{36}\pi$	0.083

Many products now contain nanoparticles. They have been used in suncreams to make them transparent. They can also be found in sports garments to make them odour-free. And they have been added as carbon fibres to strengthen car tyres and body panels. Developments in nanomedicine include the creation of nanoelectric biosystems, nanoparticle contrast agents to enhance radiological imaging, drug delivery systems in pharmacology,[16] and cell repair mechanisms in disease and trauma.

One of the most intriguing claims concerns the use of nanorobots in medicine. These tiny molecular machines would, for instance, have no difficulty navigating the narrow lumens of capillary blood vessels to carry out repair work. Already, stealthy nanoparticles have been used to invade cancer cells.

Yet predicting the medical, health and environmental impact of the nanoworld is difficult because many of the effects are unknown at present. The field is moving extremely rapidly and needs to be closely monitored.[17]

According to a report by the Royal Commission on Environmental Pollution, there are several areas that are already a cause for concern. For example, nanoparticles of silver are much more toxic than larger pieces of the metal itself, because of the huge surface contact area. When impregnated clothing is washed, these particles will inevitably enter the water supply. Sewage treatment plants rely on bacteria to purify the water. The tiny particles are more toxic to bacteria than bleach and may upset the balance. Again, carbon nanofibres, used instead of dyes for colouring in clothing, could be released into the atmosphere and inhaled. Furthermore, 'buckyballs', football-shaped nanoparticles of carbon, named after the architect Buckminster Fuller, could be absorbed by bacteria and enter the food chain.

Apart from the unknown environmental hazards of any new technology, nanomedicine has sparked speculation of a doomsday catastrophe in the realm of science fiction. The most bizarre is the 'Grey Goo' prediction. This foresees an end-of-the-world scenario involving nanotechnology, in which self-replicating molecular robots, out of control, consume all the matter on Earth, leaving only a gigantic gooey mass. Fortunately, Eric Drexler, the American engineer who predicted that nanoparticles could run amok, consuming the planet's resources, has had an 'agonising reappraisal' and now says this is highly unlikely.

Futurologists have always been around, from H G Wells to George Orwell. But Kenneth Clark, in *Civilisation*, was sceptical. He said, 'We have no idea where we are going, and sweeping confident generalisations about the future are intellectually the most disreputable of all forms of public utterance. The scientists best qualified to talk have kept their mouths shut.' The Bard agreed in *Macbeth*: 'If you can look into the seeds of time, and say which grain will grow and which will not, speak then unto me.'

Biogenesis

Any account of progress in scientific medicine inevitably leads to a discussion of biogenesis and the origin of life. Modern cosmology grapples with the mysteries of the universe and the emergence of life. Studies in evolutionary biology contribute to our understanding of disease, especially malignant disease. In the distant past, following the Big Bang, a fortuitous concourse of atoms somehow evolved into galaxies, solar systems, planets and life itself. Order emerged out of chaos.

The theory of complexity attempts to explain how this occurred. At the edge of chaos, simple atoms reshuffled themselves endlessly in a random chaotic manner. Eventually, given enough time, some complex molecules emerged. These complex molecules then locked onto similar molecules through common bonds. As the process continued, self-recognition led to self-organization. Gradually, with increasing complexity, life emerged out of the primordial soup. Some believe that the transition was triggered by a 'divine spark' in a universe that was calibrated for life's existence. Others disagree (see below).

Whatever force created life out of inanimate matter, it was the biologist William Hamilton who then explained how single cells combined to form multi-celled organisms. He called this process 'kin selection'. The term had been coined earlier by John Maynard Smith, but it was Hamilton who developed the concept: 'Nearby cells tend to be related through shared genes, so increasing co-operation made evolutionary sense.' This genetic kinship led to stronger ties between cells, which eventually congregated into tissues, organ systems and complex forms of life.

At a higher level, self-recognition and kin selection give new meaning to the proverb, 'Birds of a feather flock together.' I believe this adage encapsulates a fundamental law of nature. One sees it at every level in biology and society, whether it be swarming insects, plagues of locusts, migrating birds, male bonding in the local golf club or youths at a rock concert. The proverb can conveniently be rephrased: molecules of a kind tend to bind, or cells of a kind tend to bind.

It transpires that some forms of cancer are the antithesis of this process. Order degenerates into chaos. Contact inhibition is lost and anarchy ensues. Cells revert to a more primitive state as they lose their ability to differentiate. The most undifferentiated or anaplastic tumours are also the most malignant. Self-recognition and kin selection are lost. Unable to bind cohesively, cancer cells spread chaotically to metastatic sites. In biology, kin selection is depicted as brotherly love between genes. In oncogeny, it is replaced by sibling rivalry. The evolutionary development of normal growth is described in the dictum, *ontogeny recapitulates phylogeny*. In malignant growth the reverse is true: *oncogeny reverts phylogeny*.

One might worry that reprogramming adult cells to create pluripotent stem cells (iPS) might induce malignancy. Fortunately, there is no evidence of this so far, but these experiments need to be carefully monitored.

Creating artificial life

In May 2010, a spectacular achievement in an American laboratory caused a stir. J Craig Venter, the entrepreneurial scientist noted for self-aggrandisement, created the first artificial life form.[18] He used yeast to assemble fragments of DNA into a very long DNA molecule. In this way, his team stitched together the four basic nucleotides – adenine, cytosine, guanine and thymine – that make up all DNA, to construct a new prosthetic genome. Venter's team then inserted this into a recipient bacterium, replacing the native DNA.[19]

The cell was then powered by the synthetic genome. The artificial DNA grew and divided, creating two daughter cells, one with the synthetic DNA and one with the natural DNA. Antibiotics then destroyed the natural DNA, leaving the synthetic DNA to multiply. All traces of the recipient bacterium were eradicated, and the synthetic DNA thrived and flourished.

The discovery was hailed as a technical tour-de-force, but not necessarily a scientific breakthrough. Nonetheless, the work has far reaching implications. Some predict that synthetic biology could create bacteria designed to perform specific tasks. For instance, bacterial factories could possibly produce clean biofuels, mop up carbon dioxide and toxic waste, or generate quantities of novel drugs and vaccines. Venter, not usually renowned for modesty, noted however that gene therapy has little chance of working in the immediate future. The downside of the discovery is more worrying, should the bacteria run amok.

Dr David King, of the Human Genetics Alert watchdog, is concerned about the dangers. He says, 'Scientists' understanding of the biology falls far short of their technical capabilities.' Professor John Sulston, the geneticist who helped sequence the human genome, has challenged Venter over plans to patent the findings. Sulston says patents would be damaging,[20] and that the private sector must not have a monopoly in this field of human endeavour. He believes that these studies belong in the public domain. No doubt, the commercial prospects of this work will mean that both the private and public sectors will continue to be involved. Meanwhile, medical care is moving away from the bedside to the laboratory, leaving the morality behind.

The future of medical research is unpredictable. Science is moving ahead so swiftly that we may be taken by surprise. We may have to wrestle with the inconceivable. Some say we are heading for a singularity (see box), a technical change so rapid that it represents a rupture in the fabric of events.

Singularity

A singularity is the end result of rapid change. Two types have been described: gravitational and technological.

The gravitational singularity is the physicist's version and involves time boundaries. For instance, in a collapsing universe, when matter converges in a 'big crunch' towards the centre of a black hole, time stops.

The technological singularity is best understood by Moore's Law. Gordon Moore noted that the number of transistors in computer hardware is doubling exponentially every two years. This cannot be sustained indefinitely, and leads to the limits of miniaturization, when the transistors contract to the size of atoms, and the system collapses.

Likewise the accelerating changes in science and medicine, suggest we may be heading for an 'intelligence explosion', culminating in instantaneous instability and a rupture in the fabric of events.

References

1. Fleming N. Rival genetic tests leave buyers confused. *The Sunday Times*, 7 September 2008.
2. Hampton OA, Den Hollander P, Miller CA, Delgado DA et al. A sequence-level map of chromosomal breakpoints in the MCF-7 breast cancer cell line yields insights into the evolution of a cancer genome. *Genome Research* 2009; **19(2)**: 167–77.
3. Henderson M. DNA sequencing for all in ten years, says pioneer. *The Times*, 24 June 2010.
4. Modified viruses attack cancer. *BBC News* and *ITN*, 23 April 2010.
5. Cypel M, Yiu M, Rubacha M et al. Functional repair of human donor lungs by IL-10 gene therapy. *Science Translational Medicine* 2009; **1**: 4ra9.
6. Warren G. Briefing: Gene cures. *The Sunday Times*, 18 April 2010.
7. Syvanen M, Kado C (editors). *Horizontal Gene Transfer*, 2nd edition. Academic Press: San Diego, 2002.
8. Lowry WS. Passive immunity against childhood cancer. *Lancet* 1974; **303**: 602–3.
9. Delaney C, Heimfeld S, Brashem-Stein C et al. Notch-mediated expansion of human cord blood progenitor cells capable of myeloid reconstruction. *Nature Medicine* 2010; **16**: 232–6.
10. Snippert HJ, Haegebarth A, Kasper M et al. *Lgr6* marks stem cells in the hair follicle that generate all cell lineages of the skin. *Science* 2010; **327**: 1385–9.
11. Scientists find 'mother' of all skin cells. *Reuters*, 11 March 2010.
12. Park A. The quest resumes – after eight years of political ostracism, stem cells are back. *Time*, 9 February 2009.
13. Park A. How the coming revolution in stem cells could save your life. *Time*, 9 February 2009.
14. Henderson M. Stem cell websites give patients false hope. *The Times*, 4 December 2008.
15. McCredie J. *Beyond Thalidomide*. London: RSM Press; 2007.
16. Henderson M. New attack on cancer with nano weapon. *The Times*, 5 November 2009.
17. Sample I. Proliferation of nanoparticles poses risk. *The Guardian,* 12 November 2008.
18. Park A. Scientist creates life. That's a good thing, right? *Time*, 20 May 2010.
19. Gibson DG, Glass JI, Lartigue C et al. Creation of a bacterial cell controlled by a chemically synthesized genome. *Science* 2010; **329**: 52–6.
20. Ghosh P. Synthetic life patents damaging. *BBC News*, 24 May 2010.

CHAPTER 23

The sequelae of success

The success of medicine has created a new set of problems. Some of these were anticipated. Others were unforeseen.

Chapter summary

- The changing pattern of disease
- The biological backlash

The changing pattern of disease

The incidence of disease is shifting under our gaze. Mitral stenosis, previously a common valvular heart disease, has largely disappeared. In the past, it was a consequence of rheumatic fever and streptococcal throat infection, now largely eradicated by antibiotics. The incidence of cardiac arrest has also diminished, partly due to the decline in smoking habits. On the other hand, cardiomyopathy, a hereditary heart condition, has surfaced, possibly due to increased awareness and detection.

The pattern of infectious disease has also changed. As already noted, tuberculosis, which had virtually disappeared in the West, has reappeared in the immigrant population. Moreover, a shift in the pattern of tropical disease is predicted with climate change.

In malignant disease, there have been changes in the causes and distribution of tumours. Cancer of the oesophagus has moved from the upper third of the gullet, where it was associated with alcohol and smoking, to the lower third, where it is related to GORD (gastro-oesophageal reflux disease), or heartburn. Alcoholism itself is increasingly seen in younger binge drinkers, with a rise in liver cirrhosis. Children as young as 10 are being admitted to hospital in an alcoholic stupor. Again, cancer of the oral cavity, previously common in older alcoholics, is now being found in younger patients, partly due to changing sexual behaviour and oral sex.

In my own field, changes in the anatomical distribution of malignant melanoma, an aggressive form of skin cancer, associated with sun exposure, have been found. These are related to changes in sartorial fashions in men and women.

Happily, however, the overall trend in the pattern of diseases is one of improvement, as medical science comes to grip with a range of conditions. Nevertheless, nature is not easily tamed, and a biological backlash is underway.

The biological backlash

The allergy epidemic

Medical advances have been accompanied by a rise in the number of patients suffering from allergies. These include allergies to food, pollen and a variety of agents. The range of provocative antigens is wide, as noted in the aphorism: 'You can be allergic to anything under the sun, including the sun.'

In an allergic reaction, the body's defence system mounts an immune response against a harmless substance, such as a peanut, a scallop or a strawberry, which it mistakenly believes to be a foreign invader. Again, the reaction may be provoked simply by the presence of a cat or a dog in the room. More worryingly, it may consist of an exaggerated response to an insult, such as a wasp sting.

Allergic symptoms vary widely, and can include swelling of the lips, a skin rash, nausea, vomiting, conjunctivitis, pain, sneezing, wheezing or an asthmatic attack. Severe reactions can lead to anaphylactic shock and death.

In addition to the increase in the prevalence of allergies, the proportion of patients with multiple allergies is increasing.[1] Moreover, there is also an increase in the severity of allergic symptoms, including anaphylaxis.

The number of allergic patients in the UK has trebled in 20 years. About 6000 patients are hospitalized every year, one-quarter with anaphylaxis. In the past, about 15% of the population suffered from an allergy. Today, the figure is close to 40%. The figures have now reached epidemic proportions.

Various reasons have been proposed for the increase in allergies. The wide range of food substances and additives available to children means that they are exposed to these agents at a younger age than previously. Climate change has been implicated – global warming has increased the level of fungal spores in the environment.

The association with eczema is thought to be significant. The excessive use of soaps and detergents may have deprived the skin of its impermeable barrier, permitting allergens to enter the body directly. Experiments with mice that develop allergic inflammation have found mutations in the gene encoding filaggrin, which normally keeps the skin barrier hydrated and intact. This 'gateway hypothesis' may account for why patients with eczema sometimes progress to develop other allergic reactions, including asthma. It has been called the atopic march.

Autoimmune disease

Allergic reactions share some features with autoimmune disease. The immune system is based on the body's ability to distinguish between self and non-self. In autoimmune disease, the body fails to recognize this distinction, and the immune response is directed against the body's own tissue. Examples include rheumatoid arthritis, biliary cirrhosis, alopecia areata (sudden onset of baldness), lupus and probably multiple sclerosis.

It is currently surmised that the increase in immunological and autoimmune diseases is due to a biological backlash against advances in hygiene and medical science, the so-called *hygiene hypothesis*. Throughout history, our bodies have evolved to deal with a level of pathogens and infectious agents. These have now largely disappeared, leaving the immune system idle. It has responded by attacking harmless elements, even the body's own tissues. Epidemiology shows that immunological and autoimmune diseases are less common in developing countries than in industrialized nations. Moreover, longitudinal studies show that as countries become more affluent, and presumably cleaner, immune disorders soar.

One of the more intriguing proposals is the use of worms to treat bowel disease. It has been noted that ulcerative colitis, Crohn's disease and irritable bowel syndrome (IBS) are less common in the underdeveloped world, where worm infestations are endemic. Some preliminary studies using worms are encouraging, but many remain to be convinced about the merits of this unorthodox approach.

Antibiotic resistance

Sometimes, scientific advances consist of two steps forward, and one step back. For instance, the discovery of antibiotics later had a downside – the emergence of drug resistance and the development of allergic reactions.

The isolation of penicillin in 1927 by Alexander Fleming marked the onset of the antibiotic era. But it was not until the 1940s that Howard Fleming and Ernest Chain realized its potential. Before that, in the 1930s, the sulphonamides initiated the antibiotic revolution. The sulpha drugs are bacteriostatic, that is they do not kill the bacteria, they compete for its vital constituents.

M&B 693, manufactured in England by May and Baker, was the first sulpha drug to be marketed. It transformed the treatment of streptococcal infections. Thousands of patients were treated with the drug, including Winston Churchill and myself. I recall receiving M&B 693, as a child with scarlet fever, along with quinine, the taste of which lingers with me to this day!

The subsequent arrival of penicillin was a quantum leap in the treatment of infectious diseases. The new antibiotics were bactericidal – they kill the bugs.

It was not long, however, before drug resistance emerged. Only four years after its commercial production, resistance to penicillin was found in *Staphylococcus aureus*. Methicillin replaced penicillin, and, by 1961, MRSA (methicillin-resistant *S. aureus*) was detected in the UK. Today, half of all *S. aureus* infections in the USA are resistant to penicillin, methicillin, tetracycline and erythromycin. The epidemic of MRSA is now a modern scourge. Later, vancomycin was effective for a time before resistance emerged. More recently, resistance has also appeared to a new class of drugs, the oxazolidinones.

Resistance in staphylococci was followed by the appearance of vancomycin-resistance among enterococci (VRE). Resistance has appeared in *Pseudomonas* and *Clostridium* species, and there are now drug-resistant strains of tuberculosis, gonorrhoea and malaria.

Resistant strains arise because of genetic mutations in bacteria. This is a form of evolution in the microworld. The same phenomenon is seen with mutating viruses, bypassing vaccination programmes. Both bacteria and viruses have simpler genetic codes than higher forms of life, and are able to modify their structure quickly. Once a new strain appears, it can easily pass on its resilience, by a process known as horizontal gene transfer. Multidrug resistance has also begun to emerge, with the appearance of the so-called superbugs. NDM-1 (New Delhi metallo-beta-lactamase-1), an enzyme conferring bacterial resistance to all known antibiotics, arrived in Britain in August 2010, carried by patients who went abroad to countries like India for treatments such as cosmetic surgery.

The process has been accelerated by the overuse and misuse of antibiotics. Drugs have entered the food chain. Of particular concern is the practice of feeding livestock antibiotics, not only to combat infection, but also to promote growth.

Various attempts have been made to resolve the problem. Bacteriophages, viruses that infect bacteria, have been recruited as therapeutic tools. Some plants that exhibit curative properties in infectious diseases have also been used. The Archaea (formerly called archaebacteria) are another promising group. These primitive microorganisms live in a wide range of habitats, including extremely hostile environments such as hydrothermal faults deep on the sea bed. It is thought that they may yield new forms of antibiotic therapy.

Unfortunately, pharmaceutical companies have less interest in antibiotics today. It has been noted that products used to treat acute conditions are less profitable than those used to treat chronic diseases.

Meanwhile, scientists have discovered a major cause not only of antibiotic resistance but also of drug resistance in cancer therapy. A group of compounds, known as ABC transporters, have the ability to evict therapeutic drugs from infected cells, rendering treatment ineffective. It may yet be possible to devise a means of reversing this process. Research workers have been trying to keep a step ahead of the pathogens. It is an open question who will win. My money is on the scientists, but others disagree and see a new plague ahead.

Survival of the unfit

Many patients now survive with debilitating diseases that would otherwise have killed them in previous centuries. One obvious advance has been the treatment of diabetes mellitus. Before the discovery of insulin, patients with juvenile diabetes (type 1) had a short lifespan. Most diabetic patients now survive for long periods, although they remain at greater risk of late-onset complications.

Meanwhile, the incidence of diabetes has soared, mostly adult-onset (type 2) diabetes. There are an estimated two million diabetic patients in the UK, and ten times that number in the USA. The causes of type 1 and type 2 diabetes are multifactorial and different, but both share an underlying genetic predisposition.

Ironically, it has been noted that this rise in the incidence of diabetes[2] may cause the first fall in life expectancy in 200 years.

There is another epidemiological quirk. Although many genetic disorders now account for a higher proportion of disease than previously, this is not necessarily because incidence has risen, but because the incidence of non-inherited disease has fallen. Heritability refers to the genetic contribution, relative to the other determinants of disease. Thus, for instance, a study of rickets in Quebec Province in Canada showed a fall in incidence, but a rise in heritability. The fall in incidence was due to better nutrition with milk supplemented with calciferol. The rise in heritability reflected the correction of the environmental deficiency (vitamin D), but the persistence of the Mendelian disorder.[3]

Teasing out the genetic element in multifactorial disorders is complex. With better management of the other causative factors, it is anticipated that the heritable component will persist and may increase. At the same time, advances in genetic engineering may help offset these developments. The isolation of rogue genes in some cases may ensure that they are not transmitted to future generations, as has happened in breast cancer with a recent patient who carried the *BRCA1* gene.

Although scientific progress will continue to outwit the biological backlash in the short term, nature will always have the last word. Built in obsolescence is the norm, and in due course it is time to move on.

References

1. Emmett S. Rise in multiple allergy patients. *BBC News*, 14 April 2009.
2. Laurence J. Diabetes may cause first fall in life expectancy for 200 years. *The Independent*, 20 October 2008
3. Jekel JF, Katz DL, Wild D, Elmore JG. *Epidemiology, Biostatistics, and Preventive Medicine*, 2nd edition. Saunders: Philadelphia, 2001.

CHAPTER 24

The biblical lifespan

'The days of our years are threescore years and ten,
And if by reason of strength they be fourscore years,
Yet is their strength labour and sorrow,
For it is soon cut off, and we fly away'
Psalm 90

If we had the same resistance to disease throughout life as we had between the ages of 16 and 17, about half of us might expect to be alive in several hundred years' time. Something happens to prevent this. We call it senescence.

Chapter summary
- The existential paradox
- Life on the edge
- Defying disability

At present, the average lifespan in both Europe and America is about 80 years, slightly more for women than men, 10 years beyond the biblical target. Interestingly, in Africa, in areas not devastated by the preventable problems of starvation, AIDS, malaria and the Ebola virus, the lifespan of many individuals is similar to that in the Western World.

Contrast this with the lives of some of the great composers in previous centuries. Schubert, Mozart, Chopin, Mendelssohn and Gershwin. All died before they were 40. But even then, those who didn't succumb to the premature diseases rampant at the time – Handel, Haydn and Monteverdi, lived into their 70s. Today, we have broken through the biblical barrier, living on for added years.

It used to be said that pneumonia was the old man's friend. Antibiotics have changed that, and enabled many to live on to develop a different set of problems.

In Japan, one-third of people over 85 have Alzheimer's disease or some other form of dementia.[1] In California, one study found that 50% of women over 90 had dementia.

A provocative paper from New Zealand, published in the *BMJ*, has suggested that prevention may not help the elderly.[2] Drugs such as statins, prescribed to combat heart disease, may simply switch the cause of death to cancer or dementia. Indeed, wags have proposed a moratorium on further research into cardiac disease, since a sudden heart attack remains the preferable mode of death for most elderly physicians.

An independent panel of experts, commissioned by government, added that attempts to encourage healthier lifestyles risk adding extra years of poor health. The report comes amid rising rates of obesity and alcohol-related diseases. It also said that many public health initiatives have focused on extending life expectancy, without ensuring quality. As an example, some of NICE's ruling on drugs, which sometimes only add a few extra months to life, are mandatory, whereas its advice on exercise, which is much more significant, is voluntary.

Many, of course, survive mentally alert into old age. The recent American Presidential candidate John McCain hardly counts as elderly. He was a sprightly 72 years. Konrad Adenauer remained Chancellor of Germany until he was 87. The Finnish composer Jean Sibelius lived to 91, although he seems to have been unproductive during his last 30 years. Perhaps he set himself too high a standard. Not so George Bernard Shaw, who was cerebrating on the world stage until 94 years. Donald Soper, mentioned earlier, was a regular at Speaker's Corner in London's Hyde Park until he was 96. My own favourite is Alistair Cooke who delivered his final 'Letter from America' on the BBC a few weeks before he died in his 96th year. Equally remarkable was Pablo Casals, the cellist, who conducted his own composition, *Hymn to the United Nations*, in New York, two months before his 95th birthday.

Less well known is Fergus Anckorn. He was shot, wounded, survived a massacre, left for dead several times, beaten, starved and tortured by the Japanese, on the infamous Burma Death Railway. Yet, at age 90, he sat through a half-hour interview on the BBC programme *Hard Talk*, and spontaneously answered questions with complete clarity about his memories, his fallen friends, his colleagues and his survival. And there are many others.

The existential paradox

We celebrate the above stories, but for many the prospect of growing old and infirm is often distressing. The increased number of elderly people raises the question of what have been euphemistically called 'end-of-life issues'.

Alice Trillin[3] coined the phrase 'the existential paradox'. We feel we are immortal, yet we know we are going to die. It is this feeling of immortality that enables us to plough ahead, in spite of the problems that sometimes beset us.

The will to survive is innate in everyone. I had a disturbing reminder of this in a terminally ill patient some years ago. According to her mother, Ellen was a beautiful young woman in every way, who never smoked or drank. Yet Ellen developed advanced cancer. I was asked to take care of her during the last phase of her illness. Every known treatment had already been tried. She became the most cachectic patient I had ever known. Finally, she was cadaverous and semiconscious.

Towards the end, her intravenous infusion came out. The nursing staff, who were extremely caring, advised me that she was unaware and it probably should not be renewed. Ellen was comatose and in no obvious discomfort. Incredibly, she lived a further week. During that time, she surfaced briefly one night, and half wondered why her drip had not been renewed, and relapsed. The day before she died, she suddenly awoke, sat up in bed and spelt it out in letters: '**I want to L.I.V.E**', then fell back unconscious. I never knew a patient who fought so hard *not* to die.

Compare this with the remarks of the Irish writer Nuala O'Faolain, quoted in her obituary in *Time* magazine.[4] She confessed that when she was diagnosed with terminal cancer in 2008, life had lost its beauty. In a tearful radio interview before she died, she said, 'There is an absolute difference between knowing that you are likely to die – let's say within the next year – and not knowing when you are going to die.'

I have already described a condition called cancer angst. It raises a question about the early detection of incurable illness in patients who otherwise feel perfectly well. Is it perhaps better not to know, and live out your days in blissful ignorance? Randy Pausch would not have agreed (see below). Yet the dilemma persists.

Life on the edge

Contrast this with those who live life on the edge. Years ago I was impressed with the exploits of Hans and Lotte Hass, scuba diving with man-eating sharks 'Under the Red Sea'. Hans and Lotte were fearless, as was their cameraman.

Again during a student ski trip in the Alps, I met an elderly doctor who told me he had had multiple cardiac problems. He showed me his morphine vial in case he got into trouble. Before setting off on a black run, he said, 'When your days are numbered, you really begin to live', and added, 'I am living on borrowed time, and I didn't borrow time to sit around.'

Later on another ski trip, I met Peter Thexton (see Figure 24.1). At the time, Peter was a 29-year-old junior doctor in London. He was an avid mountaineer, having climbed many peaks, including Everest. He and his colleagues trained in the English Lake District at weekends, driving up from London on a Friday night. They kept each other awake in the car by 'revving the conversation'.

Peter related how, on a previous climb in the Himalayas, as medical officer he stayed behind with a friend who had a minor ailment. On recovery, they set out

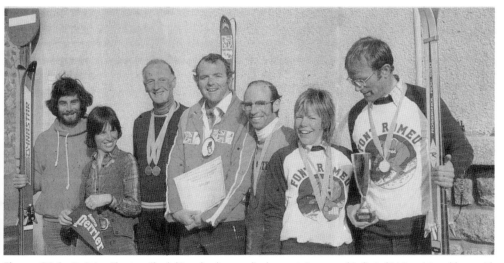

Figure 24.1 *Dr Peter Thexton (far left), a fearless medical mountaineer, on his first ski trip, pictured here with colleagues.*

to catch the others higher up the mountain. Unfortunately, on fording a waterfall, his colleague was trapped by a falling boulder in a flooded stream. Peter tried to extract the climber from the rising water, but it was impossible and the man drowned in his arms.

Peter certainly was not afraid. Although he had never skied before, on our trip he set off head first down a black run, tumbling over himself again and again, arriving at the bottom of the slope with a big grin on his face.

He told me that on his next climb, he had agreed to be the doctor on an ascent of K2, sponsored by the *Observer* newspaper. I never met him again, but years later I met the doctor who organized our ski vacation, David Delvin. I asked him about Peter. 'Did you not know?' David said, 'Peter was killed on that climb on K2.'

More recently, I spoke to Dr Clare O'Leary, a young Irish consultant gastroenterologist, and adventurer. Clare has climbed Mount Everest, and the summits on all seven continents. She has also walked to the North Pole, and next plans to do the South Pole. I asked her if she ever thought about the risks. 'Never', she said.

A man who faced tragedy with humour and dignity deserves special mention. His name was Randy Pausch, a young college lecturer in America. Randy was diagnosed with incurable pancreatic cancer in 2008. He gave his Last Lecture before a large audience. It was captured on the Internet on YouTube. The lecture was designed for all ages, but especially young people, and is entitled 'Really Achieving Your Childhood Dreams'. Pausch begins his talk by showing how fit he is. He lies down on the platform, in spite of his condition, and performs one-arm press-ups in front of the audience. A remarkable and moving confrontation with the inevitable. He died the following year.

Defying disability

How far can we extend life beyond the present biblical limits? Human beings are remarkable. Take Stephen Hawking, the physicist with motor neurone disease; Oscar Pistorius, the sprinter with artificial legs; Philippe Croizon, the French amputee, whose limbs were amputated in an electrical accident, and swam the English Channel; or Jean-Dominique Bauby, the quadriplegic journalist, who wrote a book, *The Diving Bell and the Butterfly*, by blinking his eyelids. Their determination to overcome disability is legendary.

Consider also the geriatric athletes: Philip Rabinowitz, now deceased, the sprinter from South Africa, who held the world record for the 100 metres in his age group. 'Flying Phil' was 100 years old at the time of his record. Or, most remarkably, the Japanese climber Yuichiro Miura who scaled Mount Everest in 2009 at the age of 75. Miura was beaten to the peak the previous day by 76-year-old Min Bahadur Sherchan from Nepal.

Eric Voyce deserves special mention. At 90, he is Britain's oldest bouncer and deals with drunks and soccer fans at the busy University of Wales social club. Voyce says, 'I am as fit as a fiddle and can cope with any problems. I would like to carry on until I am 100.'

over 70, those moderately overweight may live longer than those of normal weight. But being *very* overweight shortened lives. It was concluded that the elderly have a different set of risks than younger people, where obesity poses a significant hazard. It was also felt that the body mass index (BMI) recommendations need to be reviewed. The authors emphasized again that physical exercise 'really matters'.

The evidence that vitamin supplements extend life is also flawed. More encouraging is the news that resveratrol, a compound found in red wine, extends life span by around 20%. And so these studies continue.

Cloning and body part replacement offers some promise. The plan to provide pensioners with own-grown tissues is intriguing. Spare parts surgery, replacing diseased organs, is an extension of transplant surgery. The dream of replacing masses of aged tissue, worn out by time and senescence, may seem far-fetched. But the search for eternal youth continues. The hope of some researchers is to stop the clock at age 50 years. But why not at age 25, and indeed why grow old at all?

The prospect of transplanting a new brain into a youthful body, cloned from one's own tissues, has been proposed, but never been achieved. If it should happen, whose brain would it be?

Bernard Shaw might have approved. He once said, 'Youth is wasted on the young.' His predecessor, Oscar Wilde, envisaged a surreal situation in *The Picture of Dorian Gray*, a man who remained untouched by a life of debauchery, while the tissue damage was transferred to his portrait.

The barrister and playwright John Mortimer grasped the absurdity. When he was dying, he summed it up with a final witticism to Kathy Lette: 'Eternity? What an awful thought', John deadpanned, 'I mean, where's it all going to end?'

Cryonics

Cold-blooded animals, or poikilotherms, can survive severe winter conditions by hibernating. Warm-blooded mammals, including humans, have been known occasionally to recover from accidental hypothermia. Cooling has also been used clinically to treat patients with subarachnoid haemorrhage.

Cryonics, or freezing organisms with liquid nitrogen, is much more controversial. Because ice damages tissues, cryonics uses glycerol derivatives to prevent icing and crystallization. Cryonic enthusiasts believe that it will eventually be possible to keep humans alive in suspended animation, and revive them at a later date. There is no evidence yet that this is possible. However, the technique has been used successfully to preserve embryos in fertility programmes (see later).

Suspended animation

Ted Williams, the Boston Red Sox sportsman, was inducted into the Baseball Hall of Fame. When he died, he was placed in biostasis through cryonic suspension. His body parts were frozen in the Alcor Life Extension Foundation in Scottsdale, Arizona. But this dream of prolonging life indefinitely, as the aviator Charles Lindbergh and others have tried, is a nightmare not a dream. Eternal life is for theologians, not physicians. A sensible target, however, is improving the quality of geriatric life. Meanwhile, the serenity prayer of Reinhold Niebuhr is apt:

Grant me the serenity to accept the things I cannot change,
Courage to change the things that should be changed,
And the wisdom to know the difference.

Immortality

We are all immortal in the sense that we can trace our origins back through dividing germ cells, not just to our human ancestors, but perhaps all the way back to the primitive Archaea on hydrothermal vents on sea beds.

Somatic body cells have a limited lifespan, and die out after about 50 divisions or so. This is known as the Hayflick limit. The mechanism may have evolved to prevent somatic cells becoming cancerous. Cancer cells manage to defy this limit. They avoid apoptosis, or programmed cell death, by producing an enzyme, telomerase, that preserves the length of the telomeres.[5] These are the little bits at the end of chromosomes, like the aglets on the ends of shoelaces, that determine ageing.[6] Cancer researchers hope eventually to produce a drug or vaccine that might eradicate telomerase.

Immortality can be achieved in the laboratory using cancer cell lines. A commonly used experimental line is called the HeLa line. It originated in the cervical cancer tissue of a poor African American woman who died in 1951, known anonymously by her pseudonym, Helen Lane. It recently transpired that her real name was Henrietta Lacks.[7] For the past 60 years, HeLa cells have been used in tens of thousands of experiments, including the production of the Salk vaccine. The cells are unique and continue to survive in laboratories around the world.*

Undifferentiated stem cells and germ cells are not affected by the Hayflick limit. They continue to divide for the lifespan of the parent organism. It is this ability to avoid senescence that makes their use so promising for organ building. The life extensionists, however, hope that the technology can be adapted so that humans will become biologically immortal.

Everyone is getting into the act, most recently nanomedicine, discussed earlier. The future has become blurred in this imaginary world. The author Michael Crichton, who sadly died at the relatively young age of 65, wrote a best-selling visionary novel, *Jurassic Park*. That is where the discussion belongs at present, in science fiction.

At the moment, the evidence suggests that human cloning may not be possible, because of a biological quirk in primates. Hundreds of attempts to clone monkeys, after the method of Dolly the sheep, have ended in failure. The controversial scientists who have claimed to clone babies have been called charlatans. We must wait and see.

---

* Henrietta Lacks' daughter Deborah learnt about her mother's posthumous contribution to research after 25 years. Prior to Obama's health care reforms, she said, 'If my mother's cells have done so much for medicine, how come the family can't afford to see doctors?'

Ageing begins at 27 years

Professor Timothy Salthouse, of the University of Virginia, takes a different view of ageing.[8] He has found that mental powers begin to deteriorate at 27, marking the start of old age. He published the results of a seven-year study of 2000 healthy volunteers aged 18–60 in the *Journal of Neurology and Aging* in 2009.[9] Salthouse used tests that are designed to detect signs of dementia. The best performances were at 22 years. Marked decline was noted at 27 years.

It did not take an academic study to tell us that the top athletic performances in sports like tennis, swimming or gymnastics are also seen in young people, often in their teens. The same is true for mental prowess. Einstein published his Special Theory of Relativity at 26 years, and Schubert's entire musical output was mostly composed in his 20s. Moreover, in obstetrics, a woman who has her first child at 30 is known as an *elderly* primigravida. Professor Salthouse's coded message to youth is 'Don't abuse yourself, it's later than you think.'

Salthouse also noted that memory stays intact until 37 years, while the abilities based on accumulated knowledge, such as vocabulary and general information, increase until 60 years. Again, this finding is not unexpected. It reflects the nature–nurture balance. Inborn traits are there from the outset, and environmental factors are present throughout life.

All agree that short-term memory declines with age, but long-term memory is less affected. Moreover, social skills and emotional intelligence may improve with ageing. Dr Peter Connolly, of the Royal College of Psychiatrists in London, and Professor John Morrison, of Mount Sinai School of Medicine in New York, note that older people draw from experience. In a word, they may acquire wisdom.[10]

I would add that there are those for whom life begins at 40. George Bernard Shaw wrote most of his plays after middle age. And Brahms was so overawed by Beethoven that he didn't write his First Symphony until he was in his 40s. The opening musical theme of Brahms' First Symphony deliberately recalls Beethoven's Ninth Choral Symphony. It was nicknamed 'Beethoven's Tenth'.

Gallows humour, poets and philosophers

Ageing has its lighter side. I recall a former radio show where the talk show host, Wilfred Pickles, interviewed a wizened old man, and asked him the secret of his longevity. 'Well', he replied, 'I smoked and drank and chased loose women all my life.' 'And how old are you?', Wilfred asked. 'Well', he croaked, 'I'll be 35 tomorrow.'

Ingmar Bergman, the Swedish film director, when he was confined to a wheelchair and losing his eyesight, said, 'Why did nobody tell me how difficult it was to get old?' He should have asked his contemporary, the film star Bette Davis. She coined the phrase, 'Growing old is not for cissies'. Irma Kurtz agrees, and describes her feelings in her book: *About Time: Growing old Disgracefully*.

Dozens of jokes feature St Peter at the Pearly Gates. Many of the great comedians had well-worn one-liners. George Burns said at his 100th birthday, 'Its very nice to be here. Its very nice to be anywhere when you are my age.' Mark Twain's quip about exercise and funerals is too well known. Woody Allen added, 'I am not afraid of dying. I just don't want to be there when it happens.' And Bob Hope teased his wife and called her church, 'Our Lady of the Cadillacs'. As he was dying, he said, 'Surprise me!' And W C Fields' epitaph is worth repeating: 'On the whole, I'd rather be in Philadelphia.'

Ozzy Osbourne, the heavy metal rock star, relates how he went to see his doctor after abusing 'heavy-duty substances' for decades.[11] 'Let me ask you a question, Mr Osbourne', his doctor said slowly, 'Why are you still alive?'

As already mentioned, there was also Pablo Casals, the cellist, who was married several times and lived until his 97th year. At the age of 80, he married his 21-year-old pupil, Marta Montanez. His other pupils were worried about possible undue exertions on their wedding night. Casals retorted, 'If the girl dies, she dies.'

Humour is a unique human trait. It has eased the pain of many troubled souls. My 99-year-old aunt, who was blind, incontinent and lying in a London nursing home, still had her marbles. She told me she had lived too long. I said 'you will be getting a telegram for your 100th birthday from the Queen soon.' She said, 'I hope there will be a cheque in it.'

The sages, poets and philosophers have all had their say. Richard Dawkins has argued with Francis Collins. John Betjeman immortalized Devonshire Street W1. Shakespeare had lots to say. Samuel Beckett, the philosopher of despair, had a twinkle in his eye.

Albert Camus had his own credo: 'I would rather go through life thinking there was a god, and finding I was wrong; than go through life thinking there was no god, and finding I was wrong.'

The French poet Paul Claude wrote on his birthday: 'Eighty years old. No eyes left. No ears, no teeth, no legs, no wind, and, when all is said and done, how astonishingly well one does without them.' But things have improved since then.

I have had my hernias repaired, cataracts removed, a splenectomy, dental implants, and now my digital hearing aid.

References

1. Morelle R. Scientists at odds over longevity. *BBC News*, 28 March 2006.
2. Mills E. Ageing is good for us. *The Sunday Times*, 16 May 2010.
3. Leake J. Girl frozen in time may hold key to ageing. *The Sunday Times*, 9 May 2010.
4. Coren G. Does eating less make you healthier? *The Times*, 30 January 2010.
5. US Trio win Nobel prize for telomerase. *Reuters*, 5 October 2009.
6. Nobel prize for chromosome find. *BBC News*, 5 October 2009.
7. Skloot R. *The Immortal Life of Henrietta Lacks*. Random House, New York, 2010.
8. Brain decline begins at age 27. *BBC News* and *The Daily Telegraph*, 16 March 2009.
9. Salthouse TA. When does age-related cognitive decline begin? *Neurobiology of Aging* 2009; **30**: 507–14.
10. Swinford S, Kerbaj R. Brain power at full flood in the silver set. *The Sunday Times*, 27 June 2010.
11. Osbourne O. The Wisdom of Oz. *The Sunday Times Magazine*, 6 June 2010.

CHAPTER 26

Malthus and the demographic shift

In the 19th century, the Reverend Thomas Malthus (1766–1834) claimed that the world population was growing in geometrical progression. He predicted that the planet would eventually be unable to sustain the growth. Population growth has continued to expand since then, although modified by birth control, pestilence, famine and warfare.

Something that Malthus did not predict has also happened, namely the growing segment of the elderly population, as a result of death control. The world's older population is now growing by about nine million each year. In many countries, the oldest segment of the population, that is those over 80 years, is the fastest-growing component. In the USA, the older population is growing more rapidly than the entire population. Moreover, the prevalence of chronic disease in older people has resulted in increased health care spending, with high rates of disability and dementia.

In the 1970s, the population of the poorest countries was doubling so rapidly that it was predicted that the world would eventually be overrun with 16 billion people. In many countries, urgent family planning programmes were introduced. In Britain in 1990, the Optimum Population Trust (OPT) launched a 'Stop At Two' pledge. Because of the brake on reproduction, it is now predicted that numbers will rise more slowly, from the present 6.1 billion, levelling out at 9.1 billion in 2050. Some say this is manageable. Others disagree. Either way, the ratio of old to young will continue to increase.

Many believe that the world population is already too high, with countries competing for scarce resources, and famine and starvation rampant in the Third World. Sir David Attenborough, the biologist and broadcaster, lends support to the OPT, and says the swelling population is behind every threat to wildlife across the globe. He says, 'I've never seen a problem that wouldn't be easier to solve with fewer people, or harder, and ultimately impossible, with more.'

> **Chapter summary**
> - Ageing populations
> - Japan and the double collapse
> - Bankrupting the health service

In Britain in 2009, the population topped 61 million. Southeast England is now Europe's most densely populated area. Over three-quarters of a million babies were born in the previous year, mostly to immigrants who themselves were not born in Britain.

The OPT think tank reckons that Britain's population ideally should be below 30 million. Studies suggest that social wellbeing, health and happiness are related to population density. North America, Australia, New Zealand and Scandinavia are close to the OPT recommended levels.

Ageing populations

Gerontologists predict that more than half of babies born today in developed countries will live until 100 years.[1] Even if health conditions do not improve, three-quarters of infants will probably survive until their 75th birthday. Already in Britain, there are more pensioners than children under 16. The improvement in life expectancy over the last century was partly due to a reduction in infant mortality, vaccination, the treatment of infectious diseases, and latterly to improvements in lifestyle and health care. Smoking, however, remains a significant health problem.

Predictions of even longer life expectancy are based on linear projections of survival data, and on a number of assumptions. Whether the linear extrapolation will continue is a matter for debate. Professor Kaare Christensen and his colleagues in Denmark and Germany say that so far there is no sign of deceleration.[2] They claim 'we are not close to a limit, and a further rise in life expectancy seems likely'.

Shakespeare's Seven Ages of Man was simplified by gerontologists into three major periods of life: childhood, adulthood and old age. Old age has now been subdivided into two stages: a third age (young old, under 85 years) and a fourth age (oldest old, over 85 years).

Sociologists have been increasingly concerned with this demographic shift. In the 1980s, Patricia Thane, a sociologist at Goldsmiths College, London, writing for the Centre for Economic Policy Research, argued that the tone of the elderly debate was excessively gloomy. Future generations of the elderly, she said, will be fitter, more independent and able to contribute to the economy.

The evidence now indicates that this is only partly true. Studies suggest that about one-third of older people remain independent, and that fraction does not change much with ageing. This is probably because the frail and disabled die first, leaving the more robust to survive. Even so, if 50% survive to become centenarians, that leaves 50% who do not. And of those who do survive, *two-thirds will not be independent and will require supportive care.*

The situation in China has been examined and is both intriguing and instructive. Rosemary Righter, an Associate Editor for *The Times*, who has worked in Asia, has drawn attention to the spectre of the demographic shift. She says, 'When people are not only having fewer babies, but are living 30–40 years longer than they did a century ago, the result is more pensioners, and fewer workers to look after them.' This is best seen in China, where she predicts an economic catastrophe.[3] 'China has given itself a rich country's problem, before it has become rich, for all its economic performance.'

She notes that within 20 years, one-third of Chinese will be over 60. 'China has compressed into a single generation, a transformation that would rock the stability of any society.' It consists of the 4–2–1 problem: one child caring for two parents, and four grandparents. Righter concludes, 'China has no choice but to grow old gracefully.' She says, 'This might not be China's century after all.'

There is an added problem in China. Because many female fetus pregnancies are aborted, there is an acute shortage of women in some regions, distorting the reproductive pattern.

Aside from China, the demographic shift has economic consequences everywhere. In Britain, many career women fall into the fertility trap. By delaying pregnancy, they have fewer children than planned. By contrast, women who have children earlier are caught in the poverty trap. The Institute for Public Policy Research (IPPR) argues that this is exacerbating the ageing of society. Although the population is rising, the think tank believes that the fall in fertility will have long-term economic consequences.

Life insurance premiums and pension plans are based on actuarial predictions of survival. Inevitably, increased longevity will affect health care, salary patterns and retirement plans. Consider also this: the first 10 or 15 years of life are unproductive. If one retires at 65 and lives on until 100, that is half a lifetime out of the workplace.

James Vaupel, the founding Director of the Max Planck Institute for Demographic Research in Germany, describes himself as a mathematical biologist. He says there are still a number of key questions. For instance, 'Which is a more important factor for health in old age, childhood or current conditions? And which is more important, money or medicine?' He says that we don't yet know. Meanwhile, there is evidence that genetic factors play an important role, especially in the very old. A study of the genomes of 1000 centenarians by Paola Sebastiani's team in Boston found 150 genetic signposts in exceptionally long-lived people.[4] Tom Kirkwood, mentioned earlier, estimates that 'genes only account for about one-quarter of the effects of ageing'. The rest is lifestyle and environmental factors.

Growing old gracefully is a noble aim. The more immediate problem in the developed world is who will pay for it.

Japan and the double collapse

The situation in Japan is instructive, and provides a glimpse of what lies ahead. Japan has the oldest population in the world, with a life expectancy of 79.59 years for men and 86.44 for women. The country celebrates this with a 'Respect for the Elderly Day'.

In Japan, and increasingly in the West, many retired people are trying to take care of very elderly relatives. Some are going under with the strain. This has been called the 'Double Collapse'. The bulk of the health budget in Japan is spent on the elderly. A new medical plan for those over 75 years has been labelled the 'Hurry Up and Die Scheme'.

The rate of change has been so rapid that the Japanese government has no clear idea of the extent of the ageing boom.[5] Statistics are in disarray, and the authorities have lost track of the number of centenarians. No one knows the whereabouts of

Fusa Furuya, officially the oldest women in Tokyo, at 113. Her daughter cannot recall seeing her mother for almost 50 years. And it has been revealed that Tokyo's 'oldest man', Sogen Kato, allegedly on the verge of his 111th birthday, has been dead for 30 years, despite still claiming social security.

Some believe that the inability and confusion are a result of Japan's economic collapse and disintegrating social system. No one has suggested that they may be a consequence of the demographic burden.

Bankrupting the health service

Eighty per cent of the health budget in the USA and the rest of the West is spent on the last two months of life. Britain has redefined the medical problems of the elderly as social problems, and passed the financial burden to the social services. But are confusion, incontinence, immobility, blindness, etc. not health and nursing problems? And if not, how about the health problems of earlier life? Are they not also social problems that impact on society?

The reason the medical problems of the elderly have been reclassified as social problems, is of course the cost. It is predicted that nursing home care will shortly reach £1000 per week in the UK. Meanwhile, the state will only take care of the indigent. The rest must pay for themselves. This may involve using up their entire life savings, selling their home, leaving them almost destitute. A school friend of mine who spent his adult life in Canada was caught in this economic trap. Confined to a nursing home with chronic illness, his nest egg depleted, he shot himself. Some advisory bodies see bankruptcy ahead for the health service.

It is a sad fact that the majority of deaths today in the Western World take place in hospitals or nursing homes. Yet most elderly people would prefer, when the time comes, to die at home. This is a major challenge. But it is mainly a challenge for society, not for medicine.

A close medical friend of mine in his 80th year was recently diagnosed with an indolent form of prostate cancer. I couldn't resist a little gallows humour myself. I said to him, the good news is you will probably live another 10 years or more. The bad news is you will probably live another 10 years or more.

References

1. Gill V. Genes predict living beyond 100. *BBC News*, 1 July 2010.
2. Christensen K, Doblhammar G, Rau R, Vaupel J. Ageing populations: the challenges ahead. *Lancet* 2009; **374**: 1196–208.
3. Righter R. China's future will be hobbled by old age. *The Times*, 3 August 2009.
4. Sebastiani P, Solovieff N, Puca A et al. Genetic signatures of exceptional longevity in humans. *Science* DOI: 10.1126/science.1190532 (published online 1 July 2010).
5. Lewis L. Hunt for centenarians who are missing, presumed alive. *The Times*, 4 August 2010.

CHAPTER 27

A time to die

The success of medicine has created a new phenomenon: increased longevity, frailty and senescence. The pursuit of a healthy retirement and a better quality of life for the elderly is an admirable goal. But because of scientific advances, some have come to expect miracles. There is a reluctance to accept the consequences of ageing. Many have yet to come to terms with the inevitable end point, and the futility of pursuing eternal youth.

The problem does not exist in the Third World. Life expectancy in underdeveloped countries is short. The immediate question in the Western World is how will society cope with the increased numbers of elderly people, and who will pay for it?

Chapter summary
- Gerontology research
- The living will
- Assisted suicide
- Euthanasia
- Self-starvation
- Care and compassion
- Funding
- Happy retirees
- Confronting mortality

The emotional debate on assisted suicide is a distraction. Those who wish to end their own lives because of incurable illness deserve our support, but they are a small part of the problem. It is the growing number of elderly demented patients that require urgent attention. Several approaches have been taken.

Gerontology research

It is generally agreed that increased emphasis should be placed on research into improving the quality of life in older people, especially in tackling the problem of Alzheimer's disease. The aim is to achieve a healthy and prolonged retirement.

What happens beyond that has rarely been discussed. Presumably, the hope is that the very old will remain relatively mobile, and then suddenly collapse and die of a heart attack, or, better, quietly expire in their sleep. But no one can guarantee a sudden exit, and it might equally be argued that research will at best postpone and prolong the natural decline of ageing and onset of disability.

The living will

Another approach in coping with an elderly and senescent population is to encourage people to make a living will. It is a curious term, almost an oxymoron, in that it is about the mode of dying, rather than living.

A living will is a document setting out a patient's wishes in advance regarding how they want to be treated, or not treated, if and when they become seriously ill, and unable to make decisions for themselves. If it is expressed in general terms, it is not legally binding. But if specific directions are included, such as no antibiotics, then it can be legally binding. Whether caregivers will follow the instructions is another matter.

So far, there has been a remarkable reluctance of people to make a living will.

When the physician, author, poet and philosopher Professor Raymond Tallis recently asked an audience of doctors and lawyers in Belfast how many had made a living will, only one person put up his hand. The ambivalence of the audience may have had something to do with the reluctance of most people to envisage their own mortality. Living wills are for other people. Curiously, American relatives tell me that many in the USA have made living wills. Are Americans more realistic, or has this something to do with an expensive and precarious health care system?

Enacting a living will is a form of voluntary euthanasia by consent. It can take a passive form, such as withholding treatment. Or it can take the more controversial active form, by withdrawing treatment already underway. Tube-feeding a patient who is brain-dead and in a permanent vegetative state presents physicians and families with a dilemma.

There is also the problem sometimes of persuading doctors and nurses to follow the patient's wishes. Physicians may be reluctant to do so, on either moral or legal grounds. I was present at a lecture by Baroness Mary Warnock, the philosopher, when she said that doctors who refused to follow patients' wishes were 'wicked'. It recalls for me a few nurses in the distant past who were reluctant to give large doses of opiates to terminally ill cancer patients, for fear it might make the patients addicted.

The debate on living wills is important, very important. But it has little impact on the main problem – the large majority of senescent patients, sitting in nursing homes, staring blankly at infinity in front of flickering black-and-white television screens. This 'Last scene of all … is second childishness.' Sadly, such patients are often like infants, incontinent and hungry. Like infants, they demand and deserve our care and attention.

Assisted suicide

The third option is to provide the means for distressed elderly people to take their own lives, if they so wish (see box). One could leave a bottle of barbiturates by the bedside.[1] Providing the means, but not actually administering it, is highly controversial. The Hemlock Society in the USA provides information for the terminally ill in case they wish to hasten death, but this has not been widely adopted.

Suicide

Any discussion of assisted suicide should first focus on the general problem of suicide. The will to live is so strong that it is difficult for most people to understand why anyone would wish to self-destruct.

Yet suicide is a significant cause of death. Over one million people worldwide commit suicide every year. According to the World Health Organization, 40% of suicides take place in China, Japan and India.

There are two main categories: suicidal *attempt* and suicidal *intent*. Suicidal *attempt* is 20 times more common than *intent*. Many patients recover. It is often associated with an overdose of tablets and is sometimes interpreted as a cry for help. It is more common in females. Those who intend to commit suicide are usually successful, and are more often males. They may resort to gunshot, hanging, or jumping from bridges, buildings or cliffs.

Not under discussion here are those who commit suicide for fanatical, religious or political reasons, such as the Japanese kamikaze pilots during the Second World War, the hunger strikers in Northern Ireland or the suicide bombers in the Middle East.

Endogenous depression, bipolar and unipolar mood disorders, and mental illness are by far the commonest causes of suicide. Suicide is also a significant cause of death in disturbed young people. The most common group, however, are elderly males over 70 years. Many of these men are depressed and unable to cope with the problems of ageing. They may be socially isolated, or overcome by advancing illness.

Exogenous factors are also sometimes involved. Victims may be impoverished, unemployed, retired, alcoholic, disgraced, divorced, childless or addicted to drugs. Curiously, war is invariably associated with a fall in the suicide rate. Perhaps, the ruminations of a potential suicide are diverted by the crisis of wartime.

By definition, suicide is a fatal illness. Most societies view it as a tragedy (see Colour Plate 5). But this has not always been the case. In the past, some countries considered suicide as a crime, or more often a sin.

I recall in Ireland some years ago, a critical article about Sweden in the *Irish Times*. It was entitled 'Unhappy Utopia' and quoted the higher suicide rate in Sweden compared with Ireland. At the time, a medical colleague in Ireland told me how he had to give evidence at the inquest of a woman who had put her head in a gas oven. The coroner's verdict was not suicide, but misadventure. Suicide in Ireland at that time was considered a mortal sin.

The philosophical, cultural, moral and ethical issues surrounding suicide are complex. Fortunately, there is evidence that attitudes to suicide are changing. Presumably, in the minds of those who contemplate suicide, death is a preferable alternative to living in misery.

Euthanasia

The fourth option is mercy killing. The word *euthanasia* is derived from the Greek, 'a good death'. This again seems to be an oxymoron, a contradiction in terms. Euthanasia is concerned with two groups of patients. First, there are those who want assistance to die, according either to a previous living will or to a request at the time. The second group of patients are those who have not left such instructions, but who are moribund and whose lives are meaningless.

Active euthanasia – that is, killing patients for whatever reason – is considered a form of murder and is illegal in Britain. It has been sanctioned with safeguards in Belgium, Luxembourg, The Netherlands, Switzerland, and some parts of the USA. The reasons for and against voluntary euthanasia are manifest. Those in favour argue that it is the only means of relieving intolerable distress in the terminally ill. Others reject the option on moral, theological and legal grounds. They add that, even with safeguards, euthanasia is open to abuse. Patients may be pressurized to consent because they have become a burden.

My own view is that the situation is relatively uncommon. During my career as an oncologist, I can think of very few cases where it might have been indicated. On the contrary, the vast majority of patients, even in extremis, want to live. That is not to say that euthanasia is never indicated.

The debate on euthanasia usually centres around a 'good death or unbearable suffering at the end of life'. Kathryn Mannix, a consultant in palliative medicine in Newcastle-upon-Tyne, challenges this narrow approach and analyses the physical symptoms and emotional factors and the spiritual journey at the end of life.[2] Palliative medicine, however, is primarily concerned with terminally ill patients, mostly with cancer, who have a limited lifespan. This is distinct from the main problem, namely, caring for those physically and mentally disabled by various chronic conditions, mostly senile dementia. Managing these patients, who often live on for many years in a doddering 'gaga' state, is a strain on the staff of nursing homes, the relatives and the patients themselves, and a huge economic burden.

Self-starvation

Voluntary refusal of food and fluid is the most disturbing option of all.[3] Because medically assisted dying is unlawful, doctors have been helping patients starve and dehydrate themselves to death. A number of physicians in Britain have formed a group called Friends at the End (FATE), to lobby for a change in the law. The group has distributed copies of a leaflet and a book entitled *A Hastened Death by Self-Denial of Food and Drink*. They emphasize that once a person has decided to stop eating and drinking, it is essential for the family and carers to support the decision, and avoid giving the patient liquids, or even ice cubes, which might prolong the suffering.

One case that I am familiar with was highlighted in a full-page article in *The Sunday Times* on 8 March 2009. Lily, not her real name, had been my mixed doubles tennis partner some years previously. Quite suddenly one day, her speech became slurred. Both she and her husband recognized the symptom immediately because a mutual friend had died of the condition – bulbar palsy, an early symptom of motor neuron disease. Lily soon became incapacitated as her condition worsened. She wanted to end it all. However, she was unable to travel to Switzerland and her doctors could not prescribe barbiturates. Wanting to end her misery, she decided to starve herself to death. As time dragged on, she became distraught. Unable to speak, but with the aid of a computer, she wrote, 'You wouldn't put a dog through this: You would put it down; you would give it a lethal injection.'

Her daughter Jenny told me that the family doctor gave palliative doses of sedatives and opiates, and this worked for a couple of weeks. Then the suffering became horrific. Lily was howling with anguish. The palliative care team upped the dosage and she drifted into a coma. It took her five further days to die. Her ending was grotesque. In all, the hunger strike lasted 25 days. A nightmare for everyone involved. *Res ipsa loquitor* – the case speaks for itself.

Care and compassion

The debate on euthanasia, however emotional, will have to be resolved eventually. But, as already noted, it is a distraction. It is the demographic shift that has to be addressed. In 2005, 16.5% of the European Union were over 65 years. It is predicted that by 2030, one-quarter of the population will be over 65.

The distinguished physician Sir William Osler, who bridged the gap between the 19th and 20th centuries, was aware of the gravity of the problem even then. He joked about it, and was bemused by Trollope's novel *The Fixed Period*, set in Britannula near New Zealand. After a fixed period, 'departures' were arranged by cremation. Osler jokingly suggested that after a contemplative period of a year, men should be 'peacefully extinguished by chloroform'.

The novelist Martin Amis, in provocative and humorous mood, raised the question again in 2010, by proposing euthanasia booths on every street corner. The booths, he said, would provide a very useful public service, because 'when you are 70, you don't feel like walking under a bus – you want something easier than that.'

Osler himself survived an earlier bout with smallpox, but went on later to duly depart this life after his threescore years and ten. Amis, at the time of writing, is still very much alive.

Jesting apart, the majority of elderly patients, however frail, are in no hurry to depart. We have to devise means to take good care of them, whatever the cost. Clearly, elderly people who are active and enjoying life – and there are many of them contributing to society – are not under discussion. It is the elderly demented folk who have lost contact with reality that we have to deal with. The thought of mass culling of this group is not only unthinkable, it is abhorrent. So the problem of coping remains. It calls for a lost quality – compassion.

Funding

The sociologist Peter Beresford emphasizes the point. He says that the clamour for assisted dying has to be placed in its proper context. We need to address the squeamishness and prurience that surround disabilities and face up to the realities of ageing and deterioration. There is a need to challenge attitudes, cultures and taboos.

End-of-life nursing care continues to be underfunded, patchy and unreliable.

Carol Sarler adds a caveat. Writing in *The Spectator*, she says there is no dignity in this Alzheimer's parade.[4] She deplores the detail that many well-known personalities provide, documenting the decline of their elderly relatives, including the incontinence and confusion. Sarler applauds Nancy Reagan's approach. When former President Ronald Reagan developed Alzheimer's disease, he issued a dignified statement of farewell, and they both retreated behind tall gates. From then on, Nancy guarded his privacy with the ferocity of a tigress. When he died 10 years later, the only pictures available still showed the familiar grin of the former film star and president.

In contrast, 40 years earlier, Winston Churchill's doctor, Lord Moran, was heavily criticized for publishing the intimate details of the old man's physical and mental decline during his final illness.

Happy retirees

Curiously, although ageing is a downhill process, it is not all gloom.[5,6] Despite worries about money, sickness and bereavements, psychologists have found that older people are often happier as they age. Laura Carstensen and Susan Charles in California say that the elderly are aware that their remaining time is shorter, and they want to make the best of it. They have learned new skills and avoid stressful situations. They are more resilient to personal criticism. The actress Jane Fonda, on reaching 71, talks of the melancholy she feels each passing autumn. But she adds that it is a transitory feeling, and she plans to live until 101. There is a downside, of course. Those with dementia and depression are anything but happy. Sadly, they account for a substantial proportion of the elderly population.

Confronting mortality

No book on medicine can ignore the subject of death. The doctor's job is to defy death, or at least postpone it as long as ethically possible. The doctor reluctantly signs the death certificate. Patients and physicians need to re-examine their attitudes to death. The debate requires a philosophical shift. Societies – that is all of us – have to understand that whereas we are on the edge of conquering premature illness through advances, we have to look beyond science. This brings us face to face with our own mortality. There is an end point.

No one really wants to live forever. It is death itself that most fear. Fukuyama, discussing the subsidiary title of his book, *The Last Man*, is saddened by what he sees: the Last Man has no higher ideals above his own health. He lives solely to prolong his existence. He is risk-averse; a weak pitiful creature scared of death. As mentioned earlier, Alice Trillin defined the existential paradox: 'We feel we are immortal, yet we know we are going to die.' She said that we need this pretence, this deception, to stay sane.

Many find comfort in religious belief. Others look elsewhere. Ernest Becker, in his book *The Denial of Death*, says, 'scepticism is a more radical experience, a more manly confrontation of potential meaninglessness than mysticism'. He adds, 'I think that taking life seriously means something such as this: that whatever man does on this planet, has to be done in the lived truth of the terror of creation, of the grotesque, of the rumble of panic underneath everything. Otherwise it is false.'

Kenneth Clark noted that Shakespeare held a similar view.[7] The Bard felt strongly about the absolute meaninglessness of life. Clark said that the human mind gained a new greatness by outstaring this emptiness.

Barbara Ehrenreich, quoted earlier, confronting her own breast cancer, said 'Why is there no room for some gracious acceptance of death, when the time comes, as it surely will.' And the author Sir Terry Pratchett, who was recently diagnosed with an early-onset form of Alzheimer's disease, says, 'We have been so successful in the past century at the art of living longer and staying alive, that we have forgotten how to die.' Again, as mentioned previously, Alice Trillin said she was astonished to find that, having eventually faced the terror of lung cancer, her life felt richer having confronted death. As it happened, Alice survived her ordeal for some time, dying 20 years later, probably from the late side effects of her treatment.

I would add that everyone has to face up to mortality, sooner or later, and must do so on their own terms. The actor Anthony Hopkins offers his personal approach. In a recent interview,[8] he said that he no longer fears failure or death, and added, 'Once you accept the fact there is nothing to fear, you drill into a primal well. I believe when we do things without fear, we can do anything. As long as you don't worry about the consequences.' Writing his memoir about his early struggle with alcoholism, Hopkins noted that he gave up drinking in 1975 and never relapsed: 'From the moment I made that decision, a very powerful thought shot into my brain – it's all over, now you can start living.'

Unfortunately, the futile pursuit of life extension and immortality is blinding many to the new problem that confronts everyone – namely, coping with the increasing numbers of older people. We have to live within the framework of our allotted lifespan. The native North American Indians have a saying: 'Tread gently on the ground; and when the time comes, move over and make way for the unborn, yet to come.'

References

1. Finlay I. Assisted suicide is fine in a perfect world. We don't live (or die) in one. *The Times*, 1 April 2009
2. Mannix K. Seeing the end of life with peace of mind. *The Times*, 24 July 2009.
3. Kate-Templeton S. Terminally ill opt for suicide by starvation. *The Sunday Times*, 8 March 2009.
4. Sarler C. There is no dignity in this Alzheimer parade. *The Spectator*, 21 February 2009.
5. Humphrys J, with Jarvis S. *The Welcome Visitor. Living Well. Dying Well.* Hodder: London, 2009.
6. Kurtz I. *About Time. Growing Old Disgracefully.* John Murray: London, 2009.
7. Clark K. *Civilisation.* Harper and Row: New York, 1969.
8. Leve A. News Review Interview. Anthony Hopkins. *The Sunday Times*, 7 February, 2010.

CHAPTER 28

A time to be born

Not content with tampering at the end of life, scientific medicine has been accused of intruding at the start of life, especially in reprogenetics. Obstetrics has merged with reproductive medicine.

Responding to pressure from the natural childbirth lobby, the NHS agreed to introduce a target to comply with a guidance document *Making Normal Birth a Reality*. But the target may be quietly dropped, as it is uninformed and not based on reliable evidence.

Epidurals have been stigmatized as abnormal by the lobby. Yet many pregnant women find them a welcome way of reducing the intense pain that often accompanies childbirth. Pain is not ennobling. Most agree that pain relief is an inalienable right for those who request it. Caesarian sections have also been stigmatized. Again the criticism is often uninformed.

Caesarean sections

Caesarean sections are usually performed when vaginal delivery would put the mother's or baby's life or health at risk.[1] There are a number of causes for the increase in C-sections. In the past, with large families, there was reluctance to embark on a series of C-sections. Now, with smaller families, there is less pressure *not* to do the procedure. Moreover, electronic monitoring of the fetal heart has enabled anomalies to be detected before delivery. In these cases, C-sections greatly reduced intrapartum deaths. Other reasons for the increase are patient-driven. Long, hard extensive labour with difficult forceps delivery is unacceptable to many mothers. Increasingly too, C-sections have been performed on request, as a lifestyle choice. But the phrase 'too posh to push' has been exaggerated, with only a tiny minority in that group.

The number of C-sections is rising worldwide. The World Health Organization has noted that many are performed without any clear medical need. The incidence is about 22–28% in developed countries, and exceptionally nearly 50%. In America, a study in August 2010 found that one-third of births were C-sections. One reason cited in the USA was that 44% of attempted vaginal deliveries were induced, a decision that is twice as likely to lead to a C-section. The medical records did not show whether the procedure was medically necessary. Other reasons included older obese mothers, bigger babies and multiple births (IVF).

The procedure has a higher mortality than vaginal delivery, but this is misleading, as many C-sections are performed for emergency reasons. On the other hand, there is lower morbidity in later life, with fewer pelvic floor problems, including prolapse. In addition, there is a much lower rate of litigation than with vaginal deliveries.

In a separate study, the birth history of 400,000 schoolchildren in Glasgow found that babies born only one week early were at greater risk of educational and health problems, including autism, attention deficit hyperactivity disorder, dyslexia, deafness and poor vision.[2] Professor Jill Pell, who led the study, said doctors and women should consider the risks of learning difficulties when thinking about a C-section. She adds that it is 'normal policy in caesareans to deliver women one week early, but if you make a decision for an elective pre-term delivery, then it has to be a balance, weighing up the risks and potential benefits.' Meanwhile, the significance of Pell's data is unclear, as she has yet to discriminate between those delivered electively at 39 weeks with normal fetuses and those delivered at 39 weeks because of maternal complications of perceived fetal compromise. Aside from caesareans, early-term births are becoming more common, because more mothers are electing to be delivered early for non-medical reasons (so-called birth scheduling).

Home births

Home births have long been debated amid concerns about their safety. In England and Wales, 2.7% of infants are born at home; in the USA, this figure is even smaller, less than 1%. But the numbers are rising in both countries.

Advocates of home birth claim that it has important health benefits compared with hospital births – fewer lacerations, fewer haemorrhages, fewer retained placentas, fewer infections. But there is a downside if complications arise. Two new studies were published in 2010,[3] one in the *American Journal of Obstetrics and Gynecology*,[4] and the other in the *British Journal of Obstetrics and Gynaecology*.[5]

The American report was a meta-analysis of many studies, led by Dr Joseph R Wax. The report found that planned home births had twice the risk of neonatal deaths (deaths at ages 1 week to 1 month) compared with hospital births, but there was no difference in perinatal deaths (shortly before or immediately after birth). Not surprisingly, Mary Lawlor, President of the National Association of Certified Professional Midwives, found the study defective and 'deeply flawed'.

The second study, from The Netherlands, led by Professor Simone Buitendijk, analysed over half a million births and found no difference in death or serious illness among either mothers or babies. The study looked at low-risk women who planned to give birth at home, and compared them with those who planned to give birth in hospital with a midwife.

Again not surprisingly, and in contrast to her American counterpart, Louise Silverton, Deputy General Secretary of the Royal College of Midwives, said that the study 'was a major step forward in showing that home is as safe as hospital, for low-risk women giving birth when support services are in place.'

The Royal College of Obstetricians and Gynaecologists gave the Dutch study a cautious welcome, provided that the infrastructure and resources are present to support such a system, and so long as facilities are available for rapid transfer by ambulance to a maternity hospital where emergencies arise.

The same reservations apply in those regions where family doctors continue to deliver infants at home.

Resolving the demarcation dispute between doctors and nurses was discussed in an earlier chapter, along with the notion of fast-tracking training programmes in the medical subspecialities. A similar approach may be indicated in dealing with the sharply divergent views of obstetricians and some midwives.

Fetal origins

The new science of fetal origins is transforming our understanding of obstetrics. Studies have found that the intrauterine environment can be as important as genetic and other factors in determining adult health patterns, ranging from obesity and hypertension to diabetes and mental illness. Prenatal exposure to toxins and stress may induce epigenetic changes. These can modify the action of genes without altering DNA. This field is expanding rapidly.

Test-tube babies

An even more intense debate is concerned with the ethics of fertility. The prospect of uterine transplants is one of the more recent developments. But the main thrust of research has been at the cellular level: in vitro fertilization (IVF).

The first test-tube baby, Louise Brown, was born in England in 1978. Louise grew up to marry Wesley Mullinder in 2004. Their son Cameron was conceived naturally in 2006. The first American IVF baby in 1981, Elizabeth Comeau, gave birth to a son, Trevor James, in August 2010. She and her husband also conceived naturally. Elizabeth endured years of publicity. She now jokes that if she hadn't conceived naturally, she might have had to live with the headline 'Test-tube baby has test-tube baby'.

IVF has since developed considerably, and is now practised worldwide. More than four million IVF births have been recorded since Louise Brown in 1978. The main objective of IVF has always been to enable subfertile couples have children. Other indications now include single parents and same-sex couples. The main cause of female infertility is increased age; other problems include polycystic ovary syndrome (PCOS) and pelvic inflammatory disease (PID). There is also evidence that fertility is falling in males. Sperm counts have been dropping in several countries. A 1992 study in Denmark found that counts had declined 50%

in 50 years. Adult mumps has long been recognized as a cause of male sterility, but other factors are also involved. They include paternal age, the increased use of hormones in the food chain, and the presence of hormone-replacement therapy (HRT) agents ending up in the water supply. There is also evidence that some cases may be due to lifestyle hazards such as recreational drugs, alcohol, smoking and cannabis. Moreover, although the oocyte or egg can repair damage, the sperm is just DNA with a tail, and cannot repair itself.

Eighty percent of couples planning children usually achieve pregnancy in one year, and about 5% within two years. But 10–15% continue to have fertility problems. It is estimated that just over one-third of these seek treatment. Simple stimulation of the ovary with drugs such as clomifene may induce ovulation, and that alone may work. For the rest, assisted reproductive technology (ART) may be tried. Several methods are used.

- *Intrauterine insemination (IUI).* Fast-moving sperm (the best) are placed directly inside the uterus using a fine probe or needle, at the time of ovulation. Ovarian stimulation may enhance the prospect of conception.
- *In vitro fertilization (IVF).* The eggs and sperm are mixed in a dish outside the body. Once fertilized, the embryo is placed in the uterus. The technique continues to be refined. The basic method involves using drugs to stimulate the ovaries to produce oocytes. Up to two embryos are transferred to the uterus at the eight-cell stage of 2–3 days, and pregnancy ensues in 25–31% cases. Again, the influence of age is evident. Younger women in their 20s have up to 38% chance of conceiving per cycle of ART, peaking at 27 years (Professor Timothy Salthouse again). At 40 years, conception falls precipitously. The couple's own eggs and sperm may be used, or donor eggs and/or sperm. If stimulation produces too many embryos, these can be frozen and kept for future use, avoiding the need to repeat the procedure. The latest freezing process is called vitrification. This is achieved by adding a cryoprotectant. The intracellular water can thus be cooled until it hardens like glass, without the formation of ice crystals. The frozen embryo is then kept in a state of suspended animation, and stored in a liquid nitrogen container at very low temperatures.
- *Intracytoplasmic sperm injection (ICSI).* A single sperm is injected directly into the cytoplasm of the egg. This advanced technique may be used where a natural barrier is preventing fertilization.
- *Gamete intrafallopian transfer (GIFT).* In this method, the eggs and sperm are not mixed in the laboratory, but collected and transferred immediately into one of the fallopian tubes, and fertilization takes place inside the body.
- *Blastocyst transfer.* If previous embryos have failed to implant, fertilized eggs may be allowed to develop for 5–6 days to the blastocyst stage, and then transferred around the time that implantation would take place naturally.
- *Assisted hatching.* The embryo has to break out of a membrane (zona pellucida) before it can attach to the wall of the womb. This membrane can be thickened and tough. The manoeuvre can be assisted by creating a tiny hole in the membrane to ease the hatching.

Freezing eggs and embryos

The first pregnancy from a *frozen* embryo occurred five years after Louise Brown, in 1983. About 20% of IVF births now result from frozen embryos. In Britain, they can be kept for 10 years, but a record time gap was set in the USA in 1995. Debbie Beasley was 45 years old when she gave birth to her daughter Laina. Laina had spent 13 years in a refrigerator as a frozen embryo. This is thought to be the longest an embryo has been frozen and resulted in a healthy baby.[6]

There is now a trend for career women to consider freezing their eggs to delay families.[7] A survey of 100 young medical students in Leeds revealed that a majority would consider storing their eggs on ice, as an insurance against later infertility. But the statistics are not encouraging. Only about 200 births from frozen eggs were recorded worldwide by 2010. Eggs are much more difficult to freeze than embryos, because they are large cells filled with water, and are more vulnerable to ice crystals. And the technique is very expensive. In New York, it runs about $10,000–15,000 to harvest and freeze the eggs, and thereafter $500 per year to store.

Hazards

There are risks involved with IVF. Ovarian hyperstimulation syndrome (OHSS), a complication of some forms of fertility medication, is reported in about one-third of patients. It is usually mild, but can be moderate or severe in 5% of cases. The main risks of IVF, however, involve multiple births. In addition to the normal risks of twinning, there are other hazards.[8]

A survey in The Netherlands found that the maternal death rate was three times higher in IVF pregnancies, than normal fertilization. Half of these deaths were in mothers expecting twins, raising concerns about implanting two embryos. The average age of the mothers was 36 in the Dutch study. In the UK, an increased maternal death rate was noted in women over 40 years. In Sweden an analysis of 26,000 IVF cases found an increased number of cancers in the offspring, and again in the Dutch study there were six times the numbers of retinoblastoma, a malignant tumour of the eye. Studies in Britain have been difficult to evaluate, as there is no good system for tracking IVF pregnancies. Even so, a growth disorder (Beckwith–Wiedemann syndrome) was more common.

Finger shortening was found in some boys conceived by ICSI, the procedure that bypasses natural selection by injecting the sperm directly into the egg. Although more ICSI infants had congenital abnormalities compared with spontaneous conception, in a Belgian study, most of these were corrected with minor surgery. There was no significant difference in cognitive or motor development.

In Denmark, women who have undergone IVF are four times more likely to have a stillborn child.[9] It is not known whether many of these problems are due to the fertility treatment itself or to other unknown factors related to the underlying infertility of the couples. Although the Danish findings were not confirmed in Sweden, experts are hoping that single-embryo transfer will reduce some of the risks.

There is also concern that IVF may increase the incidence of obesity, hypertension and diabetes in later life.[10] These risks remain unproven, but Professor Carmen

Sapienza's team at Temple University in Philadelphia suggest that altered oxygen levels in the culture media used to keep embryos alive may alter gene expression in IVF infants (see the discussion of epigenetics earlier).

In a further development, Dr André van Steirteghem in Belgium, who co-invented ICSI, warned that the procedure was being overused, exposing patients to needless risk and expense.

In summary, it must be said that the hazards appear to be small, but nonetheless real for those involved. The results of long-term follow-up of children 'conceived in a dish' are still being evaluated. The majority of the millions of babies born through fertility treatment are still under the age of 30.

Gender selection

Surprising as it may seem, some societies place a higher value on male children rather than females. The widespread practice in India of aborting female fetuses was described as a national shame by Prime Minister Manmohan Singh in 2008.[11] Before having ultrasound in India, pregnant women must now sign a consent form agreeing not to know the sex of their unborn child. Doctors who disclose the sex can be imprisoned for up to five years. But the law is widely flouted. Describing the practice as inhuman and uncivilized, the prime minister called for a crackdown on doctors who illegally disclose the sex to parents in advance.

It is now possible, however, to select the sex of your child through in vitro fertilization. Two methods have been used, based on the fact that males have one X and one Y chromosome while females have two X chromosomes. The Y chromosome swims faster and is smaller than the X chromosome, and the two can be distinguished using flow cytometry before conception. The second method involves testing the embryos for the X and Y chromosomes before implantation. There is a small risk that the technique may damage embryos.

Sperm sorting is ethically preferable to some couples, in that the sex is decided at conception, and precludes the question of discarding an unwanted embryo. These techniques are expensive and not widely available. Gender selection is legal in the USA and Russia, but is only permitted in Britain to avoid inherited genetic disorders. One clinic in California claims to be the largest gender selection service in the world. The same group is considering allowing parents choose the traits of their unborn child, such as eye colour or hair type.

Fortunately, many pregnant women do not wish to know the sex of their unborn infant in advance, preferring to wait until the delivery to discover whether it is a boy or a girl. Tampering with the sexual distribution of the population in nature is ethically unacceptable to many people. It has, of course, been a widespread practice in farms for decades. This is something George Orwell didn't pursue in his book *Animal Farm*.

Prenatal genetic diagnosis (PGD)

The practice of embryo screening for genetic disorders is also advancing rapidly. Amniocentesis was the first reliable test for prenatal diagnosis, and has been available for over 50 years. It is not without risk, and involves taking a small sample of the amniotic fluid surrounding the fetus and submitting it for laboratory analysis. In this way, it is possible to determine whether there is a chromosome abnormality, such as Down syndrome or Edwards syndrome.

In recent years, many women are delaying pregnancy, and late motherhood has led to a 50% increase in Down pregnancies. Yet because of prenatal screening, many of these pregnancies have been terminated, and the number of Down babies has not changed.

Pre-implantation genetic screening (PGS)

Advances in IVF now make it possible to check for genetic abnormalities before implantation, thereby avoiding abortion. Aneuploidy screening allows one to determine if the correct number of chromosomes are present beforehand. The sensitivity of the testing has been refined to such an extent that it now is possible to screen for a variety of single-gene disorders such as cystic fibrosis, haemophilia, Huntington's disease and muscular dystrophy.

The first cancer-free designer baby was born in London in 2009. The baby's father carried the breast cancer gene *BRCA1*. Eleven embryos were harvested. Six of these contained the defective gene and were discarded, thereby eliminating the hereditary abnormality in that family. The evolutionary implications of this are self-evident. Killer genes are one thing, but breeding children for the colour of their eyes, intellect or prowess at sport raises the spectre of eugenics.

Consider this: *Ivy League eggs and Oxbridge sperm: no diversity. A world of nouveau wasps; ay, there's the sting.*

Further advances

In a recent development, primitive human sperm and eggs, and the germ cells that make them, have been created from embryonic stem cells. Professor Renee Reijo Pera, in California, has identified a cocktail of proteins that can coax embryonic stem cells to form germ cells. The technique offers the prospect of creating sperm and eggs in the laboratory.[12] Infertile couples could then have their own genetic children, without recourse to donors. The prospect of enhancing fertility with this technique is still some distance away.

In another development, scientists have successfully created embryos from three parents: a man and two women.[13] The technique is known as cytoplasmic transfer. The aim is to prevent damaged DNA in mitochondria, the batteries that power cells, from being passed on. The nuclei from the father's sperm and the mother's egg, which contain the parents' DNA were removed, leaving behind the faulty mitochondria. These nuclei were then inserted into a donor egg from which the nucleus had been removed, but which retained its healthy mitochondria. Professor Doug Turnbull says that it is like changing the battery on a laptop. The hope is that it will eliminate a range of rare inherited diseases, including blindness and heart and liver failure. It is, nonetheless, introducing mitochondrial DNA from a third party, and ethics campaigners say that it is another step towards human cloning. Again, research is moving ahead so rapidly that the science is getting ahead of the ethics.

Multiple births

It has been known for some time that IVF infants have a higher risk of defects and diseases outlined above. It has now been discovered that their DNA is different from that of other children. The changes are not in the genes themselves, but in the mechanisms that switch them on and off. This is due to differences in methylation, the process whereby methyl groups are attached to genes, to shut them down when they are not required. This is epigenetics and was discussed earlier. It is not known whether these changes were triggered by the IVF technology or were already present in infertile couples. One worry is that the changes could be transmitted horizontally through the gene pool to future generations.

The main complication of IVF remains the risk of multiple births. It has always been recognized that the birth of twins doubles the risk of obstetric and neonatal complications. Not surprisingly, in IVF, the number of offspring is directly related to the number of embryos transferred. In many countries, this is strictly controlled. One or two is often appropriate.

A major controversy erupted in California in 2009.[14] Nadya Suleman delivered a complete set of octuplets, all of whom were born alive. The delivery involved 46 medical personnel. It transpired that Nadya was a single parent, living with her mother in a three-bedroom house. She already had six children and was living on food stamps, welfare and a disability income.

Nadya had attended Dr Michael Kamrava. Six embryos were transferred from previous IVF treatments. Two split into twins, resulting in eight babies. One state senator from Georgia, Ralph Hudgens, was outraged. He said, 'It's unforgivable. This woman already has six children. She is unemployed. She is going to have 14 children on the backs of taxpayers. The cost of raising these children has been estimated as between one and two million dollars.

Many feel that some measure is required to rein in the lucrative baby-making business, more concerned with success rates and profit than with ethics. Jesse Reynolds, a policy analyst for the Center for Genetics and Society, says that it is an unregulated three-billion dollar fertility industry driven by money.

The medical board of California and the American Society of Reproductive Medicine are examining the case to see if there was a violation of the standard of care. Dr Kamrava is also alleged to have given fertility treatment to a 49-year-old woman who was uninsured, hospitalized and five months pregnant with quadruplets. He transferred at least seven embryos.

Costs

IVF is a commercial enterprise, and the commodity is expensive. The average price for a course of treatment in the US in 2003 was $12,400. Some have been known to pay up to $100,000. It seems surprising that couples will pay this for a hit-and-miss procedure that only has a 30–40% chance of success. Yet the urge to procreate is so strong that many will keep trying, whatever the cost.

There are, of course, other alternatives. The surrogate mother is one possibility, especially as artificial insemination (AI) has done away with the problem of an illicit sexual arrangement. Moreover, embryo adoption allows parents to distinguish between 'breeder mothers' and gestational mothers. And if all else fails, there is always old-fashioned adoption, although even here there is a shortage, and most of the would-be parents have to look overseas.

Donor dilemmas

The vexed question of donor anonymity continues to cause controversy. Anonymity is guaranteed in America. In the UK, all IVF births are registered and the identity was protected from 1991. This was reversed in 2005, and the donor's name and details are now recorded, and can be revealed when the child is 18. The change was not retroactive. But it has meant a drop in the number of donors. The profile of sperm donors has moved from students looking for a few laughs to older men, often with families of their own. Not all donors wish to know the identity of their potential offspring. The same applies to the children themselves; some want to trace their genetic background; some do not. Many, however, are keen to search for their half-siblings. Again, not all parents tell the children of their origin. This taboo subject has been compared to earlier attitudes to adoption. Meanwhile, there have been calls to renew the anonymity rule.

Because of a shortage of donors in Britain, infertile women have been going abroad for IVF (see Colour Plate 6). Some of the overseas clinics are poorly regulated, producing more multiple births and complications. For many years, it was standard practice in the UK *not* to pay sperm donors. Expenses were permitted but limited to £55 per day and a maximum of £250. This has been challenged. Women donors have to be examined and investigated, and undergo a course of injections and minor surgical intervention. They deserve some compensation. It has been proposed that they, along with sperm donors, should now get up to £800. About 2000 infants are delivered in Britain each year using donor eggs or sperm. There is concern that increasing payments will commercialize egg harvesting, undermining the principle of donation. Moreover, the dubious practice of paying donors recalls the earlier problem with blood transfusion in some countries. Drug addicts and impoverished others were donating blood for cash. Sadly, many of those transfused contracted hepatitis and AIDS.

In a recent case in the USA, a sperm donor passed on a potentially lethal heart condition, hypertrophic cardiomyopathy.[15] He was unaware that he carried the genetic defect. His sperm had been used to father 22 children. Sixteen of the offspring were traced: nine had the faulty gene, one died, and two had already developed heart disease. In a second case in The Netherlands, a sperm donor fathered 18 children through artificial insemination. He was later found to be carrying a brain disorder, known as cerebellar ataxia. The children all have a 50/50 chance of developing the condition

In the USA, there is no cap on payments and no limit on the number of donations. An intelligent attractive college graduate can get $25,000 for her eggs. One Ivy League donor was allegedly offered twice that. Some claim that young women are being exploited, and not fully informed of the risks involved. The Center for Bioethics and Culture in 2010 produced a documentary film entititled *Eggsploitation*. It states that adverts for egg donors in college magazines and campus bulletin boards violate guidelines. But the guidelines are vague and regulation minimal. There is the added problem that half-siblings may unwittingly live in the same neighbourhood because the mothers went to the same fertility clinic.

Single parents and same-sex couples can now conceive children using anonymous sperm. Under new laws in Britain, they will be able to name almost any other adult as their child's second parent on the birth certificate. A man named as the father, or even a woman as the second parent, will not need to be biologically related to the baby, and will not even need to be the mother's 'special friend' or partner. They will, of course, have to agree to accept the legal responsibility.

These guidelines were approved by the Human Fertilisation and Embryology Authority (HFEA). Critics say that the changes further dismantle the traditional family. David Jones, Professor of Bioethics at St Mary's University College in London, said, 'These fathers are more like godparents.' He added, 'It sounds like social engineering on the hoof.' Opponents say that the laws allow single women to choose random people, and will lead to false genetic information on the birth certificate. *The Sunday Times* headlined the proposals: 'Who's the daddy? Anyone you care to name'.[16]

The number of single mothers has trebled in the last 30 years, and now accounts for 20% of mothers in the UK. Some fathers on the fringe flout convention and are unconcerned with the IVF debate. One unemployed 25-year-old father, who sleeps around recklessly, is known as 'the jobless Casanova of Tyneside, England.[17] He will shortly have fifteen children by fourteen different women, and is costing the state £2 million.' (*The Sunday Times*, September 2010). On the other hand, if he had donated his sperm through a sperm bank, he might have earned up to $15 \times £800 = £12,000$.

Fertility ethics

IVF has ignited a fierce ethical debate in a number of areas, especially in an overpopulated world. There is wide variation in the availability of IVF. The UK, which pioneered the procedure, has 66 clinics, Spain 200 and Japan 600. What is acceptable varies from country to country. Catholic countries have strict controls on the use of embryos. Some academics argue that the economic contributions of those born through IVF greatly outweigh the costs of treatment. Others disagree.

The medical profession is at the centre of the debate. Some bizarre practices have emerged. In Britain, an infertility clinic raffled a human egg in 2010,[18] with free treatment worth £20,000, in a bid to open up a transatlantic trade for childless British couples. The woman can pick an egg donor from an online catalogue. Those using the service will be able to circumvent the ban in Britain on paying and preselecting donors, provided that the embryo is implanted in America.

Ethical dilemmas abound. In two cases, deaf couples sought to have deaf children to join their 'linguistic minority'. In other cases, parents have chosen to have a baby to save the life of an existing child with a rare blood disorder, so-called 'saviour siblings'. Tissue-matched embryos have been bred to provide compatible healthy umbilical cord stem cells for bone marrow transplantation.

The changes in fertility technology also mean that women in their seventh decade can become pregnant (see box). Embryos can be frozen indefinitely. In theory, a present-day Mozart, Shakespeare or Marie Curie could reproduce offspring a generation later.

Genetic engineering is tampering with nature's own evolutionary checks and balances. Alternatively, one might argue that we ourselves are part of nature, and our intervention is part of that evolutionary process. Whether this is ultimately good or bad remains to be seen. No doubt, as in other areas, the technology will be used and abused.

A puzzling paradox has been noted by the HFEA. A number of women who have had IVF treatment have changed their minds and had abortions. Up to 80 cases are being reported in Britain each year. They have decided not to become mothers for various reasons. For some, overcoming the problem of infertility has been a goal in itself. Ann Widdecombe, the former Tory minister, said women who terminated pregnancies for non-medical reasons were treating their babies like designer goods.[19]

There is one area of reproductive technology that is worrying. That is cloning. The field overlaps with stem cell technology discussed earlier. The prospect of cloning a human being is disturbing. Some freakish scientists have claimed that this has already happened, but have produced no evidence. Most agree, however, that it will happen eventually. Even more worrying is the grotesque prospect of crossing species, creating a half man, half beast, the centaur of Greek mythology.

Future trends

What of the future of reproductive medicine? Research is moving ahead so rapidly that the HFEA is unable to keep up, and has been doing a number of U-turns.

The demand for IVF has literally and metaphorically become a growth industry.[20] Concern has been expressed about the commercial aspects of selling children as commodities. Some form of political and regulatory control is essential. But the international aspects of the trade make this difficult. Some celebrities ignore national borders and treat children like luxury goods. The IVF traders argue, 'We don't sell babies. We sell care to infertile couples. We sell a process, not an outcome.' Well said, but they rarely add that the outcome has a very low success rate.

An eminent biologist, Robert Sinsheimer, said, 'For the first time a living creature understands its origin, and can design its future.'[21] Francis Fukuyama, whose work prompted the title of this book, says, 'When the genetic lottery is replaced by choice, we open up a new avenue, along which human beings can compete, one that threatens to increase the disparity between the top and the bottom of the social hierarchy.' He calls it GenRich and GenPoor.[20]

My own view is that some of these concerns have been exaggerated. There has always been disparity in breeding. Like folk tend to marry like folk. Birds of a feather not only flock together, they procreate together. Indeed, some societies have been arranging marriages for generations. In any event, only 10–15% of the population are infertile, and only one-third of these resort to ART. And ART itself has a low success rate; in addition, not all the offspring are perfectly healthy. So, although the impact is real, it is relatively small.

Looking ahead, where are we going? Could surrogate mothers be replaced by surrogate bubbles, doing away with pregnancy itself? We have already done the difficult bit, and eliminated sex and normal childbirth. The impossible takes a little longer.

In the world of reprogenetics, the physician's role is changing. This is a field where the expertise lies with the microgeneticist, and the doctor must defer to the scientist. Yes, it calls for background knowledge of the anatomy of the female pelvis, and the clinical science of hormonal manipulation. But fast-track training in this area, combining the two disciplines, is conceivable (pun unintended) – a hybrid specialist for hybrid times. This is perhaps another case for the 'dentalization' of medicine discussed earlier.

Culture shock

Beyond the fertility debate is a cultural shift. We live in a quick-fix society. Infertility is not an illness. But it is a perfect candidate for disease mongering; another opportunity for medicalizing discontent. Wedlock is no longer the bedrock of society; illegitimate children are no longer outcasts. No one need be childless.

But not all want to have children, or indeed are suited to become parents. And they too can be stigmatized. Some have deplored those couples who refuse to have children at all. Lord Sacks, Britain's Chief Rabbi, claims that Europe is dying, because its secular population is too selfish to have children.[22] He says that parenthood involves massive sacrifice of money, attention, time and emotional energy. He adds, 'It is one of the unsayable truths of our time. We are undergoing the moral equivalent of climate change, and no one is talking about it.' He noted that wherever you turn today – Jewish, Christian or Muslim – the more religious the community, the larger on average are the families.

Sacks is concerned that secular Europe is at risk, because its moral relativism could be defeated easily by fundamentalists. He made his remarks at a meeting in 2009 sponsored by Theos, the public theology think tank. He concluded, 'In a head to head contest between a moral relativist and a fundamentalist, who wins? The fundamentalist must win because he is sure he is right, and you are not sure he is wrong.'

As for only-children being spoiled, selfish and lonely, Sacks might be surprised to find that an essay in *Time* magazine in July 2010 says that this is a myth:[23] 'In fact they're just fine – and on the rise.' But others disagree. Professor Laura Padilla-Walker from Brigham State University in Utah notes that siblings promote happiness.

Postscript

A furious theological debate continues over the question of abortion, especially in Ireland and other Catholic countries. In America, the pro-life, pro-choice discussion has taken on a political dimension, even more than arguments over guns and homicide. At the end of 2009, the US House of Representatives passed the Stupak anti-choice amendment to the Health Reform Bill. The clause takes abortion rights away, even from women who have private insurance. Once again, the obstetrician is caught in the middle.

Geriatric fertility

Senior fertility doctors in Britain rejected calls in 2010 for a ban on women over 50 receiving fertility treatment, after it emerged that a 59-year-old woman was trying to obtain IVF at a private clinic.

An editorial in the London *Times* cautions, 'When the parent is a mother who will be pocketing child benefit at the same time she is collecting her free bus pass, it is understandable ... that questions will be asked.'

Maria del Carmen Bousada, a single mother in Spain, became the world's oldest mother at the age of 66 in 2006. She sold her house in Cadiz to raise the $58,000 fees for IVF in California. Maria died of cancer 2½ years later, after giving birth to twins. The *Times* asks, 'Is it fair to court such a high risk of leaving orphans to face the world? Or leave society to pick up the potential costs? Should a school child have to tend an ailing elderly mother, when the care should be in the opposite direction?'

As noted above, the fertility industry is unregulated and driven by money. This is sadly true of several other aspects of medicine. In this connection, medicine is often no different to commerce and needs to be controlled. The writer Barbara Ehrenreich notes that one greedy Wall Street financier allegedly boasted before he went bankrupt, 'When you are worth $500 million, how can you be wrong? You are God.' In private medicine, as in commerce, you cannot take money out of the equation.

References

1. Rose D, Rumbelow H. Caesarean births 'myth' demolished. *The Times*, 29 June 2010
2. Blake H. Babies born a week early at greater risk of autism. *The Daily Telegraph*, 9 June 2010.
3. Zhang J, Troendle J, Reddy UM et al. Contemporary cesarean delivery practice in the United States. *American Journal of Obstetrics and Gynecology* 2010; **206**: 326e1–e10.
4. Bakalar N. Home birth may add a wrinkle. *The New York Times*, 9 July 2010.
5. Home births as safe as hospital. *BBC News*, 15 April 2010.
6. Longest-frozen embryo is born. *BBC News*, 6 July 2005.
7. Henderson M. Career women may freeze eggs to delay families. *The Times*, 27 June 2010.
8. Leake J. IVF babies have a higher disease risk. *The Sunday Times*, 3 January 2010.
9. Smith R. Concerns raised over IVF stillbirth risk. *The Daily Telegraph*, 24 February 2010.
10. Sample I. IVF may raise risk of diabetes, hypertension and cancer in later life. *The Guardian*, 22 February 2010.

11. Gentleman A. Indian prime minister denounces abortion of females. *The New York Times*, 29 April 2008.

12. Henderson M. Scientists 'five years away' from creating human sperm and eggs in laboratory. *The Times*, 29 October 2009.

13. Walsh F. Early hopes for three-way IVF. *BBC News*, 23 April 2010.

14. McCaffrey S. Octuplets case inspires bills in at least two states to curb number of embryo implants. *Associated Press*, 4 March 2009.

15. Smith R. Sperm donor passes ailment to nine children. *The Daily Telegraph*, 30 October 2009

16. Kate-Templeton S. Mothers face crackdown on epidural births. Who is the IVF daddy? Anyone you care to name. *The Sunday Times*, 1 March, 2009.

17. Dowling K. The jobless Casanova of Tyneside. *The Sunday Times*, 19 September 2010.

18. Rogers L. Infertility clinic to raffle egg. *The Sunday Times*, 14 March 2010.

19. Rogers L. Scandal of aborted IVF babies. *The Sunday Times*, 6 June 2010.

20. Spar DL. *The Baby Business*. Harvard Business School Press, Boston, 2006.

21. Sinsheimer R. The prospect of designed genetic change. Engineering Science April 1969; **32**: 8, 13.

22. Beckford M. Europe is dying 'because couples too selfish to have children'. *The Daily Telegraph*, 6 November 2009.

23. Sandler L. The only child: debunking the myths. *Time*, 19 July 2010.

CHAPTER 29

Health hysteria

The great secret of doctors, known only to their wives, but still hidden from the public, is that most things get better by themselves; most things in fact are better in the morning.
Lewis Thomas

Health care is one of the biggest industries in the Western World. A silent conspiracy of vested interests, including equipment manufacturers, pharmaceutical companies, health personnel and others, is involved in persuading people that they need all these extra services to stay alive. It has led to a rise in the worried well and an undercurrent of health

Chapter summary
- Technology and the market place
- Residual problems
- Ease and disease

hysteria. It has also pushed the costs of health care sky high. And, as already noted by Elliott Fisher in the Dartmouth study, one-third of this care is not helping people.

Yet the concept of health 'rights' has become so entrenched in the population that any talk of rationing provokes protests.[1] This was highlighted in the USA in 2009, when the Preventative Services Task Force caused outrage by recommending that women under 50 should not undergo routine mammography. This sparked anger among breast cancer survivors, health professionals, and a range of bodies including the American Cancer Society, the American College of Radiology and the National Cancer Institute. Never mind that the report was derived from an evidence-based analysis, compiled by 16 independent experts in prevention and primary care, and was supported by the National Breast Cancer Coalition. Indeed, the report added that the radiation risks of yearly mammography in younger women outweighed the benefits.

Patient advocate Naomi Freundlich of HealthBeat, writes that Dr Carol H Lee, chair of the American College of Radiology (ACR) Breast Imaging Commission, launched a blistering attack on the Task Force recommendations, calling them 'unfounded' and 'incredibly flawed' and will 'result in many needless deaths', and added, 'they seem to reflect a conscious decision to ration care'. Freundlich notes that Lee's organization has reason to worry. The ACR estimates that $3.3 billion was spent on mammograms in the last year alone.

Cooler heads have noted that there are exceptions to any recommendation. For instance, younger women who are at higher risk because of family history certainly need to be screened at regular intervals.

Barbara Ehrenreich draws attention to the wider problem of those who insist on a positive spin on everything.[2] As a breast cancer patient, she was dismayed to hear fellow sufferers claim to love their cancer. One said, 'If I had to do it over, would I want breast cancer? Absolutely.' Ehrenreich believes that this is accentuating the positive to the point of insanity. 'Prostate cancer is an opportunity', droned another charlatan, 'It is a path, a model, a paradigm.' 'No', says Ehrenreich, 'It's a tumor!'

Elsewhere, Lance Armstrong was quoted as saying that cancer was the best thing that ever happened to him. Taken in the context of his remarkable achievements, the comment is understandable. But Armstrong had no ordinary cancer. Germ cell tumours are in a totally different category to the solid cancers of the pancreas and the lung. The treatment of germ cell testicular cancer is arguably the most successful for any tumour in the oncology textbook. I recall losing only one patient in my career, and that was before the onset of the platinum compounds.

The spirit of optimism all began simply enough with Norman Vincent Peale and his book *The Power of Positive Thinking*. Years ago, I met Peale, heard him preach, and bought a signed copy of his book. It was only later that I heard Adlai Stevenson, the US Presidential candidate, speaking at the University of Virginia say, 'I find St Paul appealing, and St Peale appalling.' Positive thinking had become fatuous optimism.

Technology and the market place

Although positive spin is less evident in the UK, protests at any form of health rationing and some of the decisions of NICE have already been noted. There is added concern about the expanding use of the Internet, and the increasing commercialization of health technology. The rise in online drug sales has also been worrying. In the USA, this has been exacerbated by direct-to-consumer advertising on television: 'Ask your doctor if this medication is for you', is interpreted as 'Challenge your doctor', or, more forcefully, 'Tell your doctor'. One might add, 'Or else!'

Bypassing the doctor began some time ago. It probably started when your body weight could be checked on the scales in the pharmacy or drug store. Before long, blood pressure could be measured in the supermarket. Then you could be checked for diabetes at a bazaar in the church hall. More recently, firms have been offering genetic profiling.

The proliferation of private laboratory tests for blood indices, tumour markers and liver function tests is now widespread. Scanning for malignant disease, aneurysms and cardiac abnormalities is now on offer in the UK from Life Line Screening, a private American health corporation. Their leaflet says 'Life Line Screening is coming to your local area.' It states, 'We could help you avoid a stroke. Vascular and Heart Rhythm Package in the UK is available for only £139. Add osteoporosis screening for an extra £10.'

Prescan UK advertises its services in the national press. It offers 'A Total Body Scan, an MOT for your body'. The accompanying literature points out that 65% of the UK population die from heart disease, strokes or cancer. It asks, 'Are you as healthy as you think you are? With Prescan, you have the possibility to check on your general state of health and live a longer and healthier life. Take control of the situation and book your personal MOT now.' The marketing trend is obvious.

Independent review groups have noted a surge in the 'worried well' calling their general practitioner for reassurance. One family doctor in Britain, Dr Jonathan Friedman, says random screening amounts to scaremongering, especially with elderly vulnerable patients. Another poll found that one-quarter of GPs had treated patients for adverse reactions to drugs bought on the Internet. More worrying is the claim that the information may be misleading, and difficult to interpret.[3] Screening tests can produce both false-positive and false-negative results.[4]

Dr John Baldwin, in Lubbock Texas, writes,[5] 'Random screening can often lead to the discovery of supposed problems that too often lead to risky treatments. This is certainly not a form of proven prevention. Nothing is more costly or more irrational than this expensive testing that has never been studied in large populations.' He was referring to an article in *USA Today* entitled 'Healthy People Do Not Need Help', which concluded that where there is no known benefit, any risk is not worth it.

Professor Christopher Hood of Oxford University, who heads the Nuffield Council on Bioethics, is concerned about the lack of regulation, but adds, 'Cutting out the GP may sometimes be a good thing, providing us with convenience, privacy and control over our health.' The Life Line Screening group claims in its promotional literature, 'Surgery, while an important treatment option, may also be avoided if risk factors are identified earlier.' So, although some of this screening is unwarranted, and may occasionally be flawed, its progress is relentless. There is no going back.

Residual problems

Medicine has evolved over the centuries. Anatomy began with cave drawings. Gradually thereafter, the gaps were filled in by various cultures. Clinical observations led to diagnoses, epidemiology and the role of simple hygiene. Huge strides were made in the 19th century as the scientific base was established. Vaccination against smallpox, mass radiography to detect tuberculosis, and mammography for breast cancer led to further progress. Therapeutic advances followed.

Traditionally, diseases have been classified into the following categories:

- congenital
- traumatic
- inflammatory
- cardiovascular
- neoplastic
- neuropsychiatric
- miscellaneous disorders

One by one, many of these problems have been isolated. Some are socio-economic, and beyond the doctor's remit. Others have been controlled either by prevention or treatment. Life expectancy is now in the 80s, but stubborn problems remain. They include pancreatic cancer, the gliomas, motor neurone disease, Parkinson's disease, macular degeneration, the psychoses and a group of others. Even so, the majority of the former causes of premature death have been eradicated, and lifespan continues to increase.

Lewis Thomas once referred to 'Half way technology – technology that is more effective than it used to be, but that is gross and ineffective compared to what it will become'. That was 30 years ago. Juggling the lifespan figures of today, I would surmise it is now better than three-quarters way technology. We are not there yet. Eternal life is not on the agenda. But the outlook is bright. Gradually, steady advances are being made. Every week brings a new discovery. At the time of writing, for instance, genes for autism and glioblastoma have been identified. It is fair to assume that many of these remaining problems will be resolved in the foreseeable future.

Ease and disease

Throughout this discussion, the gradation between health and disease has been noted. Osteopenia merges with osteoporosis. Mental illness is often a spectrum of disorders. Normal blood pressure blends into hypertension. Metabolic conditions, gastrointestinal disorders and heart disease all have varying shades of intensity. Even cancer progresses from in situ premalignancy to invasive disease. Indeed, there is a rare condition, paradoxically known as benign metastasizing thyroid carcinoma, in which patients with the condition in a Mayo Clinic study lived longer than those without the disease. Ageing marks the slow decline of vision, hearing and memory. When does a nuisance become an illness? Prevention plays a part in slowing the slide into disease. Intervention is trickier. Handling the grey zone between ease and disease is a task beyond medicine. It calls for a different approach, a philosophical shift.

Undoubtedly, unforeseen problems will appear. Yet, as Thomas also observed, the majority of illnesses that we have to face are self-limiting.[6] We are remarkably resilient. The problems we will confront in the future may not be medical. They could be the age-old problems created by ourselves: social conflict, corruption, brutality, trauma and warfare. Add to that famine and pestilence. And behind it all is the elephant in the room: overpopulation.

References

1. The uproar over new breast cancer screening guidelines. Barbara Ehrenreich's blog, 2 December 2009.
2. Ehrenreich B. Smile or die: how positive thinking fooled America and the world. *Granta*, January 2010.
3. Fears over web health revolution. *BBC News*, 20 April 2009.
4. Warning over private health scans. *BBC News*, 2 May 2009.
5. Baldwin JC. Scans carry more risk than benefit. *USA Today*, 3 May 2010.
6. Thomas L. The technology of medicine. In: *The Lives of a Cell: Notes of a Biology Watcher*. Viking Press: New York, 1974: 35–42.

Chapter 30

The final furlong

Between my finger and my thumb
The squat pen rests.
I'll dig with it.
Seamus Heaney

The end of a chapter

One may ask, how can medicine be finished, given that we are spending more on health care than ever before? The answer is that health care is no longer about medicine; it has become something else. The job of medicine has been to eradicate premature disease. That task is almost finished and the focus has moved on. Life expectancy has expanded into the 80s. The new goal is immortality or life extension. Health care is now a colossal commercial enterprise, promoting investigations, medications and longevity. Most of the health budget is spent during the last few months of life, trying to push the limits back. *That is where the money is.*

This is the end of medicine as we have known it, the end of a chapter. There have been other chapters in the history of medicine. But this time there is a difference. Medicine is being off-loaded – 'outsourced' is the buzz term – to the physician assistant, the nurse practitioner, the technician, the administrator and his targets, and ultimately the machine. Patients no longer want to be examined. They want a PSA (prostate-specific antigen), or an MRI (magnetic resonance imaging). Soon they will want a graphic of their genome. The profession has been robbed of its personality. The doctor no longer knows best. Only the machine knows the diagnosis.

The physician is now a provider, and the patient a client. In the new marketplace, the customer is always right. Compassion has been lost in the process. No one can argue that more precision, more accurate diagnosis is a retrograde step. The new problem is often one of over-diagnosis. This in turn can lead to over-treatment. In addition, we are beginning to pick up problems we can do little about.

In the pursuit of perfect health, we must not forget that our bodies are machines. Like all machines with moving parts, after decades of use and abuse, we begin to run down. For we all have biological flaws in our protoplasm. Built-in obsolescence is the norm. It has a medical name, apoptosis. In due course, we are programmed to move on from this world. As for the scanner, it has no humanity. It is unconcerned.

The last doctor

Are we then approaching a science fiction scenario? Can we envisage doing away with physicians altogether? The Internet has rendered many activities redundant. Look what has happened to the music industry as people download tracks and concerts. Consider the demise of newspapers, as readers turn to the Internet. Take travel agents. Many people now make their own travel arrangements on the web. In the same way, patients increasingly check the computer for medical information. It is conceivable for one to make a diagnosis on the computer, and arrange the medication accordingly. Even surgery is entering the robotic age.

An example of web diagnosis was reported in the UK in February 2010.[1] Carly Hornbuckle was told that her four-year old daughter Bella had nothing serious, and was probably 'attention seeking' following the arrival of her baby sister Imogen. Not satisfied, the worried mother fed the child's symptoms into a search engine. Back came the result. All the symptoms pointed to a brain tumour. A brain scan confirmed the diagnosis of a rare condition, medulloblastoma. Surgery, radiation and chemotherapy followed. Interestingly, I used to treat this condition with radiotherapy, and this too can now be managed by computerized technology.

The process of outsourcing medicine began some time ago. Consider what has happened almost silently over the years. Take anatomy and physiology. Formerly, these subjects were taught by medical graduates. Today, these teachers have mostly been replaced by PhD graduates. Consider also what has happened, and is happening, as nursing merges seamlessly into medicine. Midwives were delivering infants long before obstetricians. In the USA, there is a distinction between anaesthetists (nurses) and anaesthesiologists (doctors). Why not smooth out these distinctions? In Russia, the demarcation line has almost disappeared. The feldsher has been acting as the country doctor for over a century. In Britain, nurses are playing an increased role, fulfilling routine medical tasks, including running clinics and meeting 'service performance imperatives'. Nurse practitioners can now safely perform intricate procedures, such as colonoscopy or OGD (oesophago-gastro-duodenoscopy), and it is only a short step to undertaking more complex manoeuvres. Above all, physician assistants in the USA have taken the final step, examining, diagnosing and treating a range of conditions. Often, they are doctors in everything but name.

The success of medicine has created a large pool of the elderly and infirm. Someone has to take care of them. But their problems are not primarily medical. They are the problems of second childhood: immobility; confusion; difficulty dressing, feeding, cleaning and bathing; falls; incontinence; and problems with communication. These are not medical problems, but nursing problems. As the need for doctors declines, the demand for nurses is increasing. By that, I mean vocational nurses, not academic administrators.

As already noted, most illnesses in middle life are self-limiting conditions – dyspepsia, headaches and febrile illnesses – that do not require skilled medical attention. The epidemic of swine flu in 2009 demonstrated that patients can often manage very well without a doctor, or even a nurse. A widespread publicity campaign advised febrile patients NOT to go to the doctor's surgery, but to stay at home, go to bed and treat themselves! Doctor substitutes and computerized technology have brought us to the point where the diagnosis and management of many conditions do not require medical involvement (see box).

The clinical supermarket

The small shopkeeper has been replaced by the supermarket. The same trend is seen in health care. The single-handed general practitioner is moving into the polyclinic. One can foresee the next step, the health care supermarket, a combination of an Internet café, medical library, electronic laboratory and health farm. Here's how the future might look, if you haven't worked it out already.

You go to the superclinic and plug into a terminal. No need for a PIN or password. It recognizes you from your fingerprint or retina. And it has your personal and family history. You pick from a menu of symptoms, and the machine directs you to the high-tech lab and superscanner. Then you either collect your product off the shelf or self-refer to the appropriate health technician or robot. If satisfaction is not forthcoming, you go to customer services for advice and re-direction.

Beyond that, the people working out at the edge on the frontiers of medicine are, by and large, not doctors. They are technologists, molecular biologists and epidemiologists. The result of a recent poll on the biggest advance ever made in medicine was not the discovery of penicillin but the discovery of X-rays, by Konrad Roentgen, a physicist. As for laboratory medicine, it is worth recalling that Louis Pasteur was not medically qualified. Godfrey Hounsfield, who invented the CT scanner, was not even a college graduate, yet went on to win the Nobel Prize in medicine. James Vaupel, who has mapped out the future lifespan of the human race, is a mathematical biologist. Craig Venter, who created artificial life, is a scientist, not a physician. And, as noted earlier, the first anaesthesiologist, William T G Morton, was a dentist.

The number of bogus doctors who have practised medicine over the years is a disturbing example of the ease with which physicians can be impersonated. Frank Abagnale, the confidence trickster depicted in the film *Catch Me If You Can*, spent nearly a year masquerading as the chief resident in paediatrics in a Georgia hospital, under the alias of Dr Frank Connors. But there were dozens of others in various countries.[2] Joanne Hartland, a research fellow at Bath University in England, identified over 100 bogus doctors, including 30 employed in the UK

National Health Service. One worked as a general practitioner in Britain for several decades. He was never suspected, and only found out when unmasked by a family member.

One way or another, medicine is slowly being eroded as it merges with para-medicine. Osteopathic medicine has been formally recognized on both sides of the Atlantic, and has shown that there are alternative routes to medical and surgical care. The physician is gradually being replaced by a melange of health professionals and doctor substitutes. This process is likely to continue, for two reasons. First, it makes evolutionary sense, with the emphasis on preventive medicine as science comes to grip with premature disease. Second, it will appeal to politicians and managers, since it is likely to save money in an age of escalating health costs. Whether it will save lives is a different debate.

Is the last doctor then a figment of the imagination? Possibly. Someone has to program the computer. In any event, who would one sue when things go wrong? What does that leave? Well it leaves surgery, or does it? Prevention is still better than the scalpel. One prominent surgeon quipped, 'Surgery is for patients, not for doctors.' Surgery has gone through the laparoscopic age, and is now entering the robotic age, the age of the technician. Does the dexterity of the surgeon require the long and arduous years of training? Maybe so, but you cannot teach a man to have good hands. It is a gift. And if Professor Salthouse is right, and our skills peak at age 22 years, and decline from 27 onwards, is it not time to move a little faster?

Take dentistry. Dental surgeons specialize in diseases of the oral cavity. They have limited medical training, yet are now involved in complex surgical procedures, including implanting prostheses into the maxilla and mandible. Dentists are not concerned with diseases of the hand or the spleen. A rudimentary background knowledge of basic medicine is all that is required, before the detailed training in dental surgery. Again, the podiatric surgeon is not medically qualified yet performs invasive surgery on the foot.

Could the same fast-track training not be applied to the diverging 57 subspecialties? The Barraquer teenagers have shown what can be achieved in ophthalmology. How about oto-rhino-laryngology, radiology, anaesthesiology, psychiatry, histopathology? The list is long. Some might say long overdue.

Already there are signs that the lengthy medical training programme may not always be necessary. A trend is emerging for fast-tracking the medical degree. As noted earlier, Texas Tech University started a three-year MD programme in September 2010, for students who want to enter family medicine.[3] Three-year medical degrees already exist in two Canadian universities. Consider again the physician assistant, trained in the medical model in two to three years. Where do you cross the line of a continuum? Fast-track training is not new to medicine. It was used to train doctors in the Second World War.

It is safe to say however, that when premature disease has been conquered, one area will remain: *trauma*. Much of trauma is self-inflicted. We have seen this on our roads. And also on the killing fields of mankind. But even in war zones, highly skilled paramedics have been transfusing patients and stitching up the wounded.

So, although the last physician is a foreseeable possibility, surgical technicians will be around for some time to come. It was prescient that the specialty in Britain retained the titular address of Mister, rather than Doctor, inherited from the bygone age of the barbers.

The end of a book

There is another sense in which we have reached the end of medicine, closer to Fukuyama's concept. Not just the end of a chapter, but the end of a book. The end of medicine as such. We are approaching the end of a moving walkway. The end of the scientific quest, the eventual triumph of medicine over premature disease. It is now up to others to take over where medicine leaves off.

This is not to minimize the stubborn problems that remain. The final problems always take a little longer to resolve. Although medicine is approaching an end point, it never quite gets there. In mathematical terms, it is an asymptote. As one nears the end of an exponential curve, the final goal always remains just out of reach. It is a law of diminishing returns.

Molecular biology has opened a new era. Although we have within us the seeds of our own destruction, we also have within us the key to our own survival. These developments promise a new era, in which health care will look very different. But it will not be an era in which the doctor holds sway. Molecular biology has unified medicine. It is also writing the final chapter.

References

1. Britten N. Mother diagnoses daughter's brain tumour from Internet research. *The Daily Telegraph*, 8 February 2010.
2. Timmins N. Dozens of bogus doctors found in health service able to fool the NHS. *The Independent*, 24 February 1996.
3. Blaney B. Texas Tech offers quicker degrees to family doctors. *Associated Press*, 24 March 2010.

CHAPTER 31

Carpe diem

Amortality

Catherine Mayer has added a footnote to the quest for immortality.[1] She has described a novel condition that she calls *amortality*. The amortals are a new group consisting mostly of baby boomers resisting the onset of age, in a time of increased life expectancy and a decline in organized religion.

Amortals, she says, 'live in the same way, at the same pitch, doing and consuming much the same things, from late teens right up until death'. She quotes Madonna and Nicolas Sarkozy as prime examples. I would add Joan Bakewell, the broadcaster; Giorgio Armani, the fashion designer, and former medical student, who has just launched a new range of fragrances at 76; and two octogenarians, Clint Eastwood, the award-winning film star and director, and André Previn, the jazz pianist, classical conductor and now opera composer.

Amortals don't just dread extinction, they deny it. Mayer says that as they age, amortals may strain the public purse, but their determination to wring every drop out of life keeps the private sector booming. They spend, whether they have money or not, they prop up the tottering music industry, they are lifelong consumers of gadgets, and they keep gyms busy, and beauty parlours and cosmetic surgeons in demand. One 90-year-old I know has just bought a new match set of golf clubs.

Mayer adds, 'From their youth, when they behave as badly as adults, to their dotage, when they behave as badly as youngsters, they refuse to be pigeonholed by age.'

For all her erudition, Mayer's concept is hardly new. Horace coined the Latin phrase *Carpe diem* – Seize the day. Again 'Eat drink and be merry, for tomorrow we die' is a conflation of two biblical sayings: *Ecclesiastes* 8, 15 and *Isaiah* 22, 13. Johannes Brahms' Academic Festival Overture is based on the mediaeval student song *Gaudeamus Igitur,* extracted from *De Brevitate Vitae* – on the shortness of life, let us rejoice.

Earlier, in the Babylonian *Epic of Gilgamesh*, Siduri tries to dissuade Gilgamesh in his quest for immortality, urging him to enjoy life as it is:

> As for you Gilgamesh, fill your belly with good things: day and night, night and day, dance and be merry, feast and rejoice. Let your clothes be fresh, bathe yourself in water, cherish the little child that holds your hand, and make your wife happy in your embrace; for this too is the lot of man.

The amortals belong to the present. They enjoy themselves. But the life extensionists, they are preoccupied with tomorrow. They have failed to learn from antiquity. Tomorrow belongs to tomorrow's children.

The life cycle

I began by saying that more has happened in science in our lifetime than in the whole of previous history. This remains true of medicine. But some things haven't changed. The theme of life and death has always been with us. Medicine is trapped in the middle. Andrew Marvell, the metaphysical poet, placed the two in juxtaposition in the poem 'To His Coy Mistress':

> The grave's a fine and private place,
> But none I think do there embrace.

In our own time, the theme persists. It was chillingly depicted in the Oscar-winning film *The Godfather*. The director, Francis Coppola, framed a shocking scene where the baptism of an infant was alternated, seemingly endlessly, with the massacre of rival gangsters by the Mob. And the theme endures on the world stage. As the global population soars, 'Why do the nations rage so furiously together?'

Conclusion: questions and answers

As medicine edges towards an end point, the profession is suffering from a severe case of future shock: *Toffler's syndrome*. Doctors have been on the back foot. We have been flying by the seat of our pants. Ad hoc-ery is the modus operandi.

Arbitrary improvization hasn't worked. We need a different approach to cope with the evolutionary changes. I hesitate to use Kuhn's well-worn term, a paradigm shift, but I cannot think of a better phrase.

Meanwhile, there is no consensus on the future role of the doctor. The finding that every living cell in the body contains all the information, in its molecular switchboard, to make an entire human being is a staggering revelation. We have no idea where we are going, or where it will end. The future is unpredictable. Some say that the accelerating change will lead to a singularity, a rupture in the fabric of human history. What is evident is that medical science is moving ahead so rapidly that it is leaving the ethics and the law behind.

Medicine has been the victim of its own success. In conclusion, it is proposed that a philosophical shift will be required by both patients and doctors to adjust to the new world. It is hoped that people will come to terms with the triumphs and limitations of the technological age, accept the reality of life and death, make the most of their active years, and the best of their sunset years.

Let me finish with a favourite story.[2] Milton Friedman, the Nobel Prize winner in economics who advised Ronald Reagan and Margaret Thatcher, invented market forces. It became known as Reaganomics. At one stage, Friedman was invited to become external examiner at Strathclyde University in Scotland. One year, the students complained that the questions he set were the same as the previous year. 'Ah yes', said Friedman, 'but the answers are different.'

The same is true for medicine. The questions are the same: Where is medicine heading? What does the future hold? But the answers are different. They no longer lie with medicine. The future of medicine is being dominated by forces outside its control. The answers now lie with sociology and economics, with bioengineering and education – the name 'doctor' means 'teacher'. Above all, the answers may lie with moral philosophy, and, dare I add, religious belief.

References

1. Mayer C. Amortality. *Time*, 12 March 2009.
2. Lowry S. Sounds familiar. Correspondence. *The Times*, 18 May 2007.

Epilogue

I have gathered a posie of other men's flowers,
and nothing but the thread that binds them is mine own
Montaigne

This book, like some other works, stands on the shoulders of those who have gone before. I would not go as far as one distinguished author, who says that all his work is plagiarism on a cosmic scale. But I would agree that much of it is a distillation of other people's work. That, if anything, is its strength, not its weakness. In drawing it all together, one hopes nonetheless to add some elements of originality.

Once a book has been published, it belongs to its readers and not to the author. For the writer, it originates as a mixture of ideas and experiences 'that he then crystallizes into a reductive try at sharing'.[1] The readers must then absorb the words and thoughts in their own minds, where they take on new shapes and meanings. I would not be surprised to see, and indeed would welcome, a response entitled *The Return of Medicine*.

References

1. Radovsky SS. Correspondence. *New England Journal of Medicine*, 1985; **313**: 1613.

Index